Manual of Equine Dermatology

This book is dedicated to my equine family, which inspires me every day to become a better person and a better veterinarian.

Manual of Equine Dermatology

Rosanna Marsella, DVM, DACVD

Department of Small Animal Clinical Sciences,
College of Veterinary, Medicine University of Florida

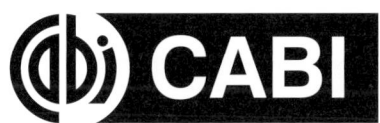

CABI is a trading name of CAB International

CABI
Nosworthy Way
Wallingford
Oxfordshire OX10 8DE
UK

CABI
745 Atlantic Avenue
8th Floor
Boston, MA 02111
USA

Tel: +44 (0)1491 832111
Fax: +44 (0)1491 833508
E-mail: info@cabi.org
Website: www.cabi.org

Tel: +1 (617)682-9015
E-mail: cabi-nao@cabi.org

A catalogue record for this book is available from the British Library, London, UK.

ISBN-13: 978 1 78639 508 5 (hardback)
          978 1 78639 509 2 (ePDF)
          978 1 78639 510 8 (ePub)

Commissioning editor: Alex Lainsbury
Editorial assistant: Tabitha Jay/Emma McCann
Production editor: Marta Patiño

Typeset by SPI, Pondicherry, India
Printed and bound in the UK by Bell & Bain Ltd, Glasgow

Contents

Preface

Dermatology is a common problem in clinical practice and can be very frustrating, as many skin diseases look somewhat similar. Thus, busy clinicians frequently end up doing symptomatic treatment rather than actually diagnosing the cause of the problem. This type of approach, although providing quick relief in the short term, tends to fail in the long term as it does not address the actual cause of the disease.

Many dermatological diseases are also chronic and progressive, leading to frustration for both the clinician and the owner, and can significantly impair the quality of life of the patient. Therefore, this book is intended to help clinicians successfully diagnose the most common skin diseases of horses. This book is not intended for dermatology specialists and its goal is not to focus on in-depth discussion of the pathogenesis of diseases unless this has a clinical relevance and direct application. The idea behind this book is to provide an easy-to-read, clinically applicable, problem-based approach to the most common dermatological presentations in equine practice for general practitioners and trainees. The goal is to provide clinicians with a *forma mentis* on how to troubleshoot dermatological diseases. Once this logical approach is learned, it can be applied to a variety of problems. The specifics may vary, but the basic rules of approach can be generalized.

This book is not intended to be inclusive of all skin conditions, nor is it intended to be categorized by mechanism of disease. Rather than present diseases by etiology, the chapters are focused on the diagnostic approach for various specific clinical presentations. Many images have been included to provide visual information on the variety of clinical presentations. Tables and flow charts also have been prepared to summarize the basics of the approach to the various problems. Each chapter has useful references that can help with additional learning when readers are interested in developing a more in-depth knowledge about specific conditions. It is hoped that, after consulting this book, when presented with a dermatological case, the clinician will have a clearer idea on how to troubleshoot the problem and develop a diagnostic and treatment plan to help equine patients.

Acknowledgements

A special thank you to all the equine patients, their owners and their referring veterinarians; as well as to my colleagues at the University of Florida, who have contributed to my exposure and knowledge in equine dermatology.

1 Approach to a Dermatological Case

Dermatological cases are common in clinical practice and can be frustrating and challenging for a variety of reasons. The most common challenge is that many diseases look alike once the initial primary lesions are replaced by secondary and less specific lesions. Taking a history is helpful to understand how the disease looked originally compared with how it presents at the time of evaluation.

Another challenge in dermatology is that the majority of cases present with some form of secondary infections and a level of pruritus. It is helpful to know whether the disease started with pruritus or whether the pruritus developed later in order to discriminate whether the itch is primary or not. It is also important to know whether the lesions were present at the very beginning or the eruption came later, or if the skin lesions are simply the result of self-trauma. All of these considerations can greatly change how the case is approached and whether a correct diagnosis is achieved or not.

The challenge for the clinician, therefore, is to separate primary from secondary symptoms and to determine what started first and what developed later. The clinician should strive to identify, if possible, the primary lesions and their distribution. Equally important is to address the secondary infections and then re-evaluate the type of lesion and pruritus that is still present to determine whether the pruritus is due to infections or to the primary underlying disease.

From the clinical standpoint, it is helpful to consider a problem-based approach when considering differential diagnoses for a dermatology patient. Once the primary lesions and their distribution have been identified, diseases that present with these lesions can be considered and ranked, based on the rest of the history. A diagnostic plan can be made to rule in or out the various differential diagnoses. The purpose of this book is to provide a problem-based approach rather than presenting diseases based on etiology or pathogenesis.

History and Signalment

When evaluating a dermatology patient, the history is crucial, as many diseases can be differentiated based on the history. One example of how the history can help discriminate among differential diagnoses is that of a horse presenting with a highly pruritic hemorrhagic lesion on its pastern in the south-eastern USA in the summer. This horse could be considered for both pythiosis (caused by *Pythium insidiosum*) and habronemiasis (caused by *Habronema* spp.). Both diseases are highly pruritic and can present with white hard granules in the exudate, commonly described as kunkers, and have many eosinophils on cytology. The course of these two diseases, however, is very different and so is the prognosis. While habronemiasis has a slow course and the patient may have had a previous history of recurrent summer sores that get better in the winter and reoccur the following summer, the pythiosis patient has a fast progression of disease that does not get better with the change of season. Knowing the speed of progression, whether the animal has had similar lesions before and the exposure to standing water can greatly help to differentiate between these two diseases, allowing a prompt diagnosis, the correct treatment, and an accurate prognosis.

Another example is a 10-year-old Warmblood horse presenting with the complaint of severe head and neck pruritus in the fall in Florida, with no prior history of pruritus reported by the owner. Allergies typically occur in young individuals but, typically, do not wait 10 years to manifest themselves in a place like Florida, so other differentials such as parasites or systemic disease should be considered. Crucial, however, is the fact that this horse lived for the first 9 years of its life in New York State and relocated to Florida only a few months ago. Thus, it is very likely that it could have allergies, possibly to *Culicoides* spp. midges, and that this is likely to be the cause of the severe pruritus in the fall.

Signalment (age, breed and sex) can help with the ranking of differential diagnoses, as some diseases are more likely to occur in the young or the elderly (e.g. dermatophytosis), while others are typical of middle-aged animals (e.g. autoimmune diseases), although exceptions are always possible. Some diseases may have a different prognosis depending on the age of the patient. For example, pemphigus foliaceus occurring in foals, typically carries a better prognosis than when it occurs in middle-aged or older horses.

Taking note of the breed can also help with the index of suspicion about certain diseases, although this information should not be extrapolated to create 'clinical blinders'. For example, draft horses are more prone to *Chorioptes* infestations than other breeds due to the presence of feathers. However, this does not mean that a pustular eruption present on the coronary band of a draft horse should automatically be assumed to be due to *Chorioptes* mites. It may very well be pemphigus foliaceus in a draft horse. Therefore, it is important to consider the presence (or not) of pruritus and to perform the appropriate tests (e.g. cytology to detect acantholytic cells) and to carry out skin scrapings to detect *Chorioptes* spp. to rule in or rule out differential diagnoses.

The history provides the clinician with important clues on where to focus during the physical examination and how to rank differential diagnoses. While some questions are standard, others may be based on the level of suspicion of the clinician and on the clinician's experience. It is always helpful to understand how the disease has changed over time, whether the animal has traveled, how long it has been owned by the current owner and where it has lived before. The purpose and lifestyle of the horse are important to know. For example, it is useful to know whether the horse is turned out and whether this is done at night or during the day, whether fly sprays are used and what kind, and how the horse has responded to previous treatments. It is relevant to know whether other concurrent diseases are present and, if so, which medications are being given. If a poor response to previous treatments is reported, it is important to double check that the doses and duration of treatments were appropriate in order to give the correct level of importance to that piece of information. For example, if a poor response to 3 days of penicillin is reported by the owners, this does not rule out pyoderma, as the appropriate course is usually at least 2 weeks.

Thus, clinicians need to develop appropriate skills on which questions to ask based on their index of suspicion, as sometimes relevant information is not freely volunteered by owners. Importantly, owners may be concerned about one problem and may be unaware that the problem is linked to something else. For example, they may be concerned about the lameness of the horse and may not be aware that the lameness is not due to an orthopedic issue but to the fact that the horse has a vascular problem and the swelling in the lower legs is painful enough to induce a reluctance to work and hence lameness. Thus, they might want radiographs done when in reality they needed a dermatology consult, and what they had underestimated as a bad case of scratches could turn out to be an immune-mediated vasculitis triggered by ultraviolet (UV) exposure.

Skin lesions evolve over time and frequently end up looking different from their original appearance. For example, owners may call the veterinarian to evaluate severe ventral edema and not mention that the horse had severe hives 2 days earlier. The edema in this case is simply the resolving stage of the severe episode of hives. Asking questions about what happened in the weeks preceding the episode of hives, such as the use of vaccines or drugs or a new batch of hay is very relevant. Often, it may not even be something that was given directly to the patient, but rather could be something that was given to another horse stabled next to the patient. As an example, for a severely groundnut-allergic horse, it is sufficient that its Timothy hay is stored in the same feed room as the groundnut hay of another horse to create cross-contamination and induce severe hives and angioedema. Asking questions about management and changes is important to pinpoint the trigger.

It is always helpful to ask how long the problem has been present and what the skin condition looked like initially. As owners are sometimes not good at describing lesions, it is helpful to ask if they have pictures or ask for the records of any other veterinarian who has examined the horse previously. It is important to ask if and how the problem has changed over time, whether it has changed slowly or rapidly, and whether any seasonality effects have been noticed.

Knowing whether other horses are affected is also relevant. If so, this may be suggestive of either a contagious disease (e.g. *Chorioptes* infestation) or a management issue. For example, if multiple horses in the same herd are itchy on their legs and ventral abdomen, this may be suggestive of mites but could also be because all of these horses are kept in the same pasture next to an area of standing water and no fly spray or deworming medication is given to the horses, placing them at risk for insect bites and onchocerciasis (caused by the parasitic worm *Onchocerca volvulus*). Skin scraping and management changes can provide some answers as well as significant relief to these horses.

The presence and distribution of pruritus is relevant, as some diseases have a peculiar distribution of lesions and pruritus. Detailed knowledge of these aspects of the dermatological presentation by the evaluating clinician is very important.

Dermatological Physical Examination

Once a general physical examination has been performed, it is important for the clinician to perform a thorough dermatological examination. The skin should be examined for loss of hair (alopecia), changes in color of both the hair and the skin, the presence of an eruption (rash), crusting, scaling, changes in thickness of the skin, the presence of draining tracts, and the presence of lumps and swellings.

Clinicians need to be familiar with both primary and secondary lesions: through an accurate physical examination to detect primary lesions and their distribution, it is possible to formulate a list of differential diagnoses. The skin has only a few ways to react, and in animals, the primary lesions are often quite short in duration. Primary lesions arise *de novo* in the skin and are a reflection of the underlying etiology. They are not always present at the time of examination, and especially not in chronic cases. Primary lesions must be looked at in relation to the whole horse, taking into account the history and their distribution. It is important that the clinician has a thorough knowledge of the different types of primary lesions. Secondary lesions are evolutionary lesions, and recognition of these and the time sequence in which they occur play an important role in allowing the clinician to formulate a differential diagnosis. Thus, the history, the presence of pruritus and the distribution of lesions are all critical factors in the ranking of differential diagnoses.

The following sections describe alopecia and changes of color, and define the different types of primary and secondary lesions. Definitions of other commonly used terms in dermatology can be found in the Glossary.

Alopecia

This is a common clinical sign in horses and may occur spontaneously or be created by self-trauma. Spontaneous hair loss is a sign of a disorder of the hair follicles, such would be seen with folliculitis or immune-mediated diseases. When hair loss is due to pruritus, the hair can be removed by a variety of means (e.g. scratching, rubbing, biting) by the animal.

There are a number of different types of alopecia:

- *Focal alopecia*: a single, small patch of alopecia (Fig. 1.1).
- *Multifocal*: multiple, small, circular patches of alopecia giving the coat a moth-eaten appearance (Fig. 1.2).
- *Regional alopecia*: affecting just one region of the body, e.g. leg.
- *Symmetrical alopecia*: the same distribution on both halves of the body.
- *Hypotrichosis*: a less than normal amount of hair (Fig. 1.3).
- *Defluxion/effluvium*: a sudden widespread loss of hair (Fig. 1.4).
- *Easy epilation*: the ability to easily remove excessive quantities of hair with little resistance; this can be due to folliculitis or a sudden shift of the hairs into the telogen phase as often occurs after a stressful event or severe illness.

Changes in color of the skin

Changes in color of the skin can be defined as follows:

- *Erythema*: skin that is redder than normal, usually suggesting the skin is inflamed. This occurs most often in allergy, in parasite and other infections, as a result of photosensitivity (Fig. 1.5) and in immune-mediated skin conditions. Erythroderma means generalized erythema.
- *Hyperpigmentation*: skin that is darker than normal. Excessive pigment in the epidermis makes the skin appear black-colored. This occurs most often with chronic skin conditions. Excessive pigment in the dermis gives a grey-blue appearance to the skin.
- *Hypopigmentation*: skin or hair that is lighter than normal. Loss of pigment can occur from hereditary, autoimmune, nutritional, neoplastic or post-inflammatory conditions (Fig. 1.6).

Primary lesions

Macule

A macule is a circumscribed, flat area of discoloration of the skin. Macules can be any color: they can be erythematous (Fig. 1.7), hemorrhagic (ecchymosis), depigmented (Fig. 1.8) or hyperpigmented.

Papule

A papule is a circumscribed elevation of skin of less than 1 cm in diameter (Fig. 1.9). Papules are always erythematous. On the body of short-coated horses, papules can be seen as tufts of hairs sticking out and may be confused with hives.

Pustule

A pustule is a circumscribed epidermal or dermal accumulation of purulent exudate (Figs 1.10 and 1.11).

It is preceded by a papule. Pustules are transient, so they quickly rupture or dry and may be mixed with secondary lesions such as crusts and epidermal collarettes.

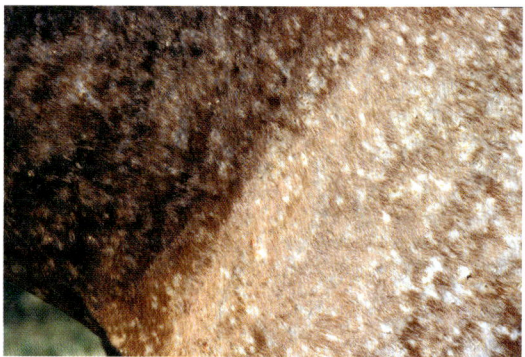

Fig. 1.2. Multifocal alopecia in a case of contact allergy.

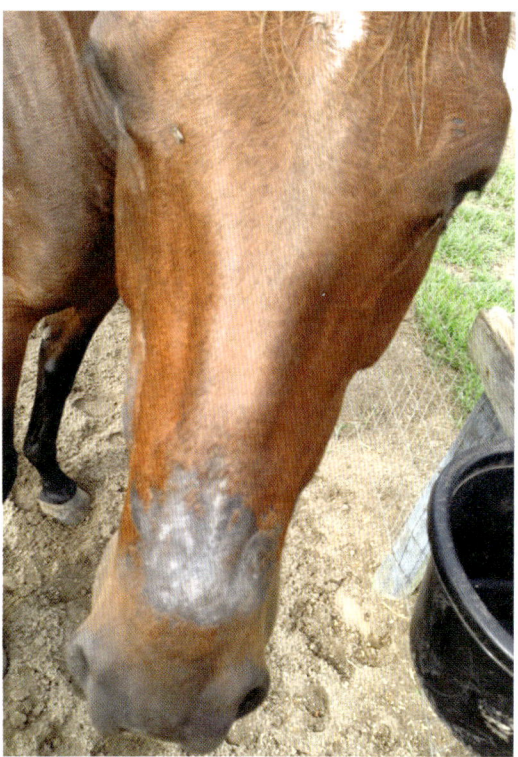

Fig. 1.1. Focal area of alopecia in a horse with dermatophytosis. The lesions were found where an infected halter had been used.

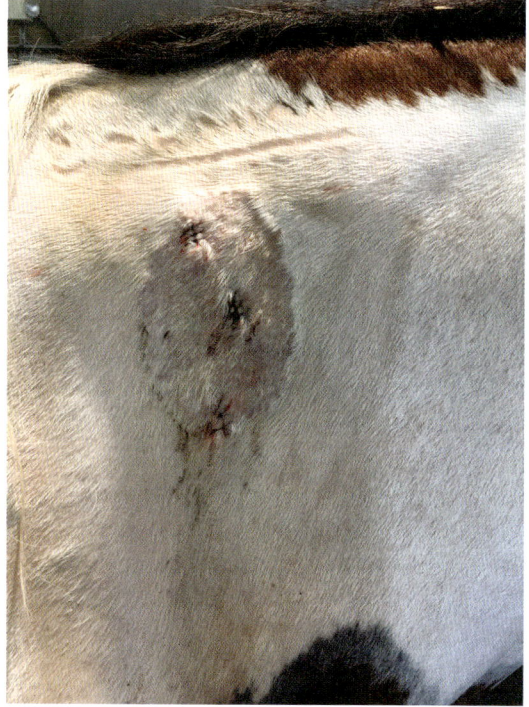

Fig. 1.3. Hypotrichosis in a horse that had developed phaeohyphomycosis infection secondary to an injection.

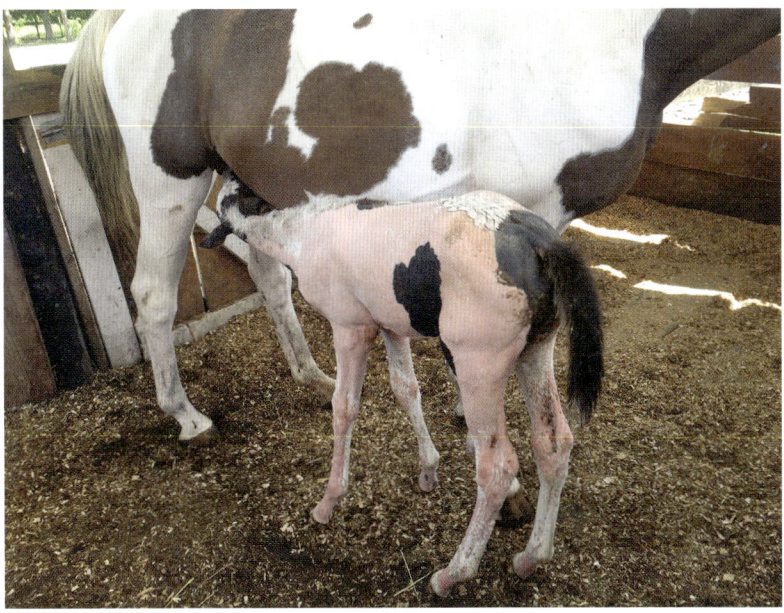

Fig. 1.4. Telogen effluvium in a young foal due to severe stress.

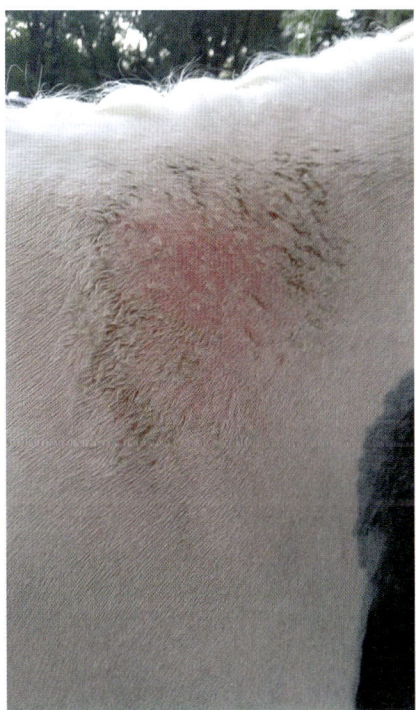

Fig. 1.5. Erythematous skin in an area with dermatophilosis, which can increase sensitivity to UV exposure, particularly evident in lightly pigmented horses.

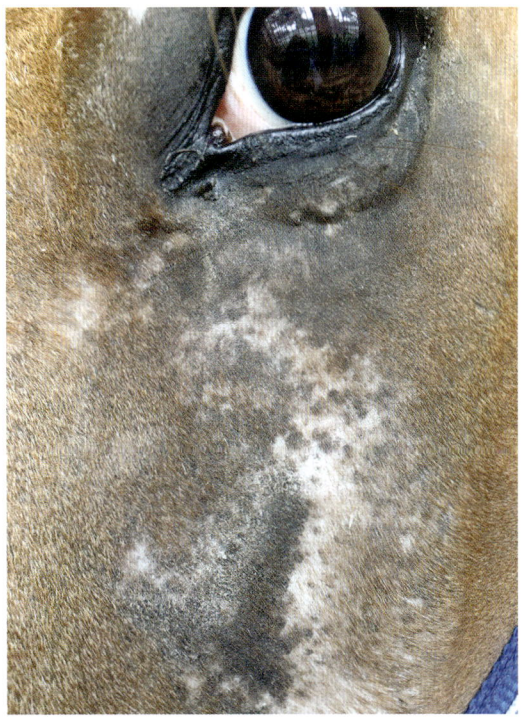

Fig. 1.6. Post-inflammatory depigmentation in a horse recovering from secondary bacterial and yeast infections.

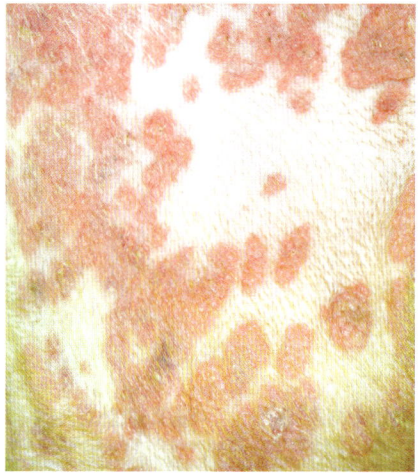

Fig. 1.7. Erythematous macules in a case of allergic reaction. The lesions are flat and red.

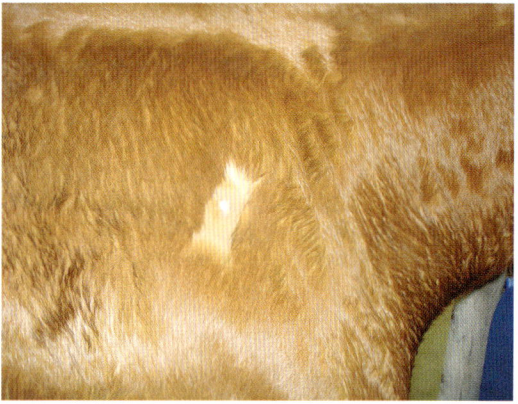

Fig. 1.8. A depigmented macule of unknown etiology

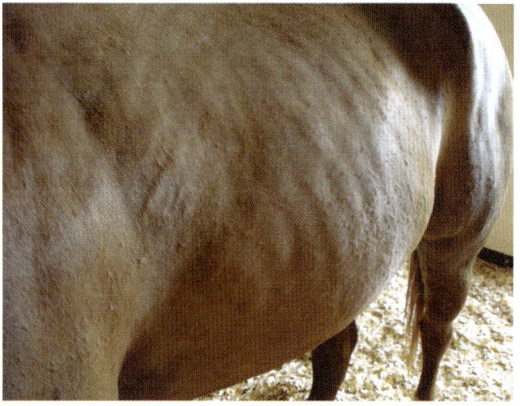

Fig. 1.9. Papular eruption in a case of staphylococcal pyoderma secondary to insect allergy.

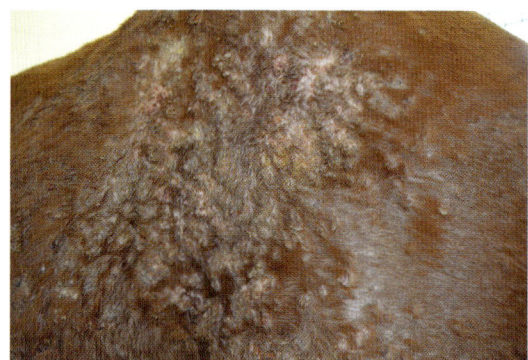

Fig. 1.10. Pustular eruption and crusts in a case of generalized staphylococcal pyoderma.

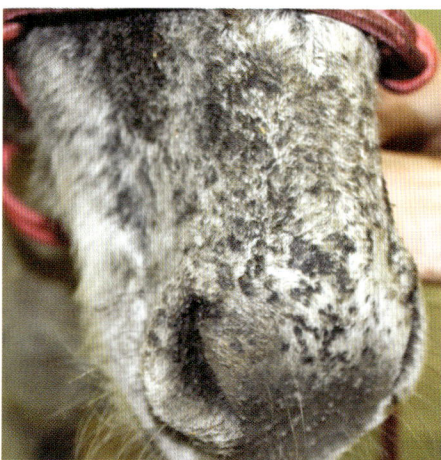

Fig. 1.11. Dry pustules and thick crusts in a case of pemphigus foliaceus. The lesions span multiple follicles and the crusts are tightly adherent to the skin.

Nodule

A nodule is a circumscribed lesion raised above the level of the epidermis (Fig. 1.12), often extending into the dermis.

Plaque

A plaque is a raised, flat-topped solid lesion (Figs 1.13 and 1.14).

Tumor

A tumor is a swelling or enlargement. It is usually, but not always, neoplastic (Fig. 1.15).

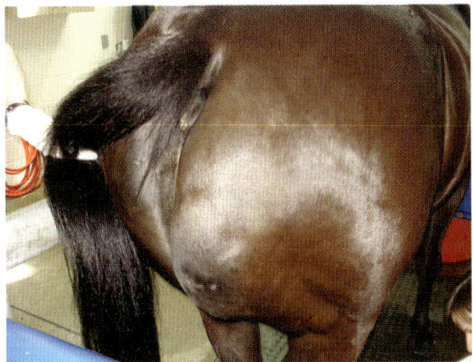

Fig. 1.12. Large nodule on the rump of a horse caused by a bacterial infection.

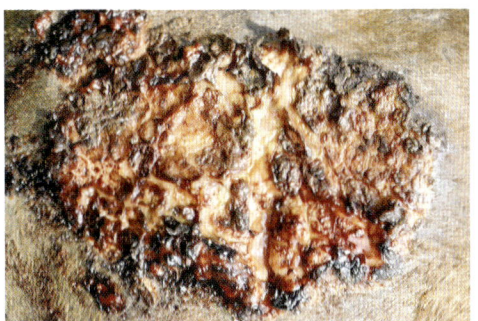

Fig. 1.13. Large plaque infected with *Habronema* sp. This area was previously a wound site. With the development of habronemiasis, proliferative ulcerated plaques have developed draining a serosanguinous exudate.

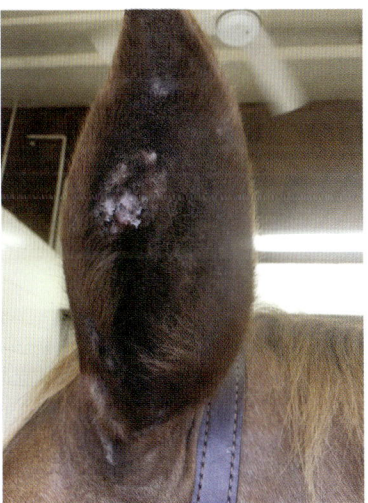

Fig. 1.14. Aural plaque on the concave surface of the pinna.

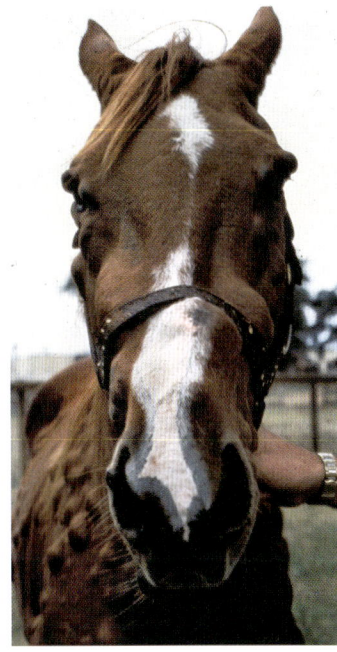

Fig. 1.15. Large tumors on the face of an older horse diagnosed with lymphoma.

Wheal

A wheal is a circumscribed skin elevation produced by edema of the superficial dermis (Figs 1.16 and 1.17). The term hives and wheals are often used interchangeably. Small hives may look like papules from a distance. One way to differentiate them is to put pressure on the skin to see whether the lesions disappear. If they do, they are hives; if they do not, they are papules. Hives are the result of vasodilation, while papules are the result of accumulation of inflammatory cells.

Vesicle

A vesicle is a circumscribed elevation of the epidermis caused by accumulation of clear fluid within or beneath the epidermis (Fig. 1.18). They are very transient and rupture easily.

Bulla

A bulla is a large vesicle formed from intraepidermal or subepidermal accumulation of serous fluid (Fig. 1.19).

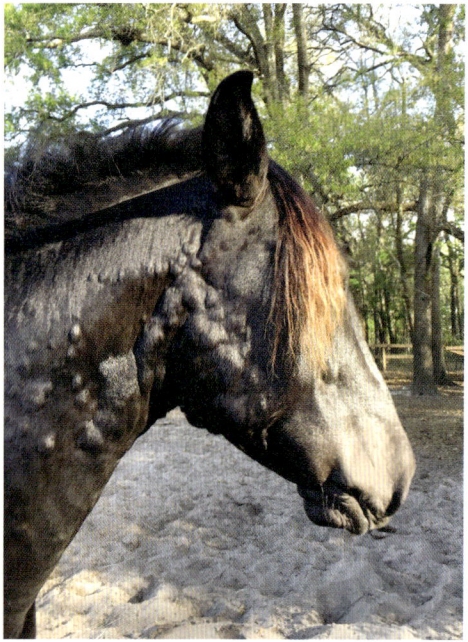

Fig. 1.16. Hives due to an allergic reaction to horse cookies. The lesions are raised and blanche upon pressure.

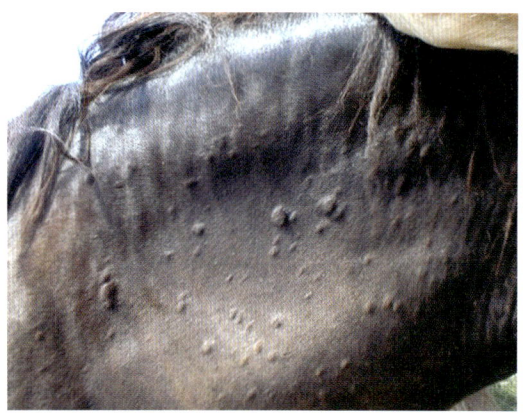

Fig. 1.17. Hives on the neck of a horse allergic to groundnut hay.

Secondary lesions (evolutionary)

Epidermal collarette

An epidermal collarette is a lesion that results from pustules coalescing, breaking and flaking off leaving a rim of flaky skin (Figs 1.20 and 1.21).

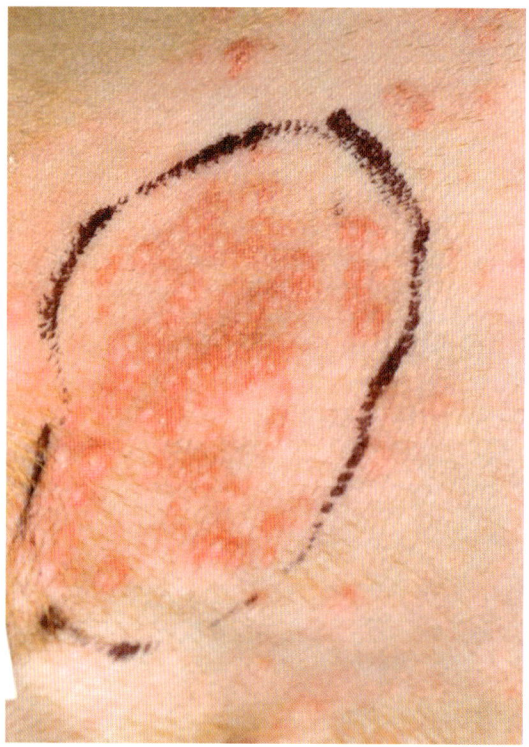

Fig. 1.18. Vesicles that developed at the site of a patch test. The lesions are filled with fluid and are very fragile.

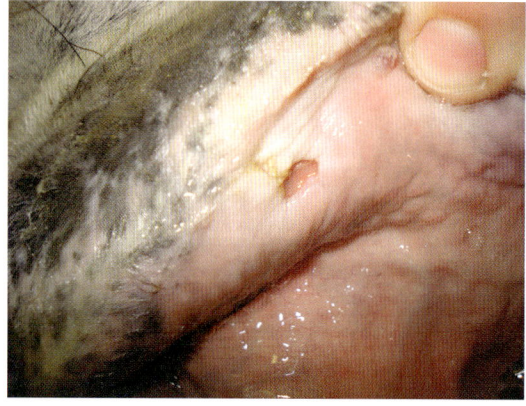

Fig. 1.19. Ulcers in the oral cavity of a horse diagnosed with bullous pemphigoid. These are secondary lesions that have evolved from the rupture of a bulla.

Crust

A crust is the dried exudate from secretion with or without epithelial or bacterial debris (Figs 1.22 and 1.23).

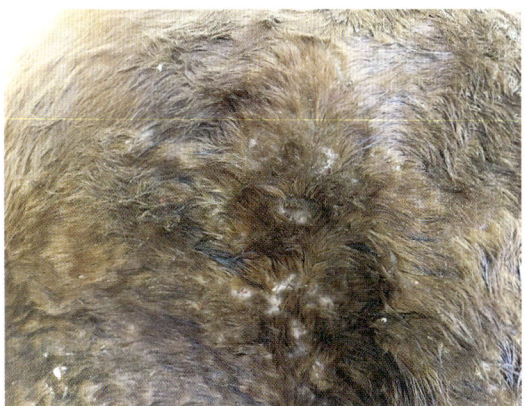

Fig. 1.20. Epidermal collarettes that have developed from the rupture of coalescing pustules in a horse with staphylococcal pyoderma.

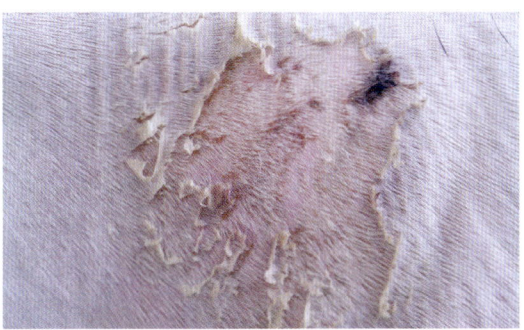

Fig. 1.21. Collarettes and exfoliation in a horse with dermatophilosis.

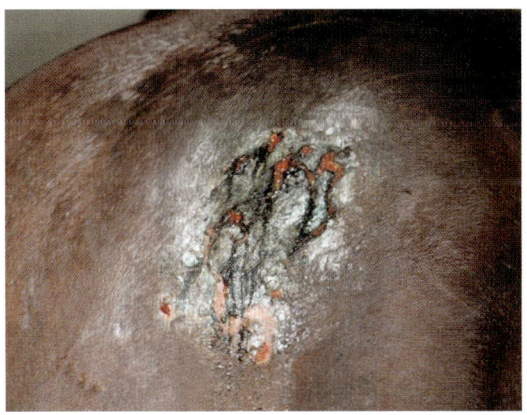

Fig. 1.22. Thick crusts and ulcers in a horse with habronemiasis.

Scales

When pustules dry and break, scales are visible in the hair (Fig. 1.24).

Scar

A scar is a fibrotic area resulting from healing of a wound or lesion (Figs 1.25 and 1.26).

Excoriation

Excoriation describes a superficial erosion or ulcer, usually caused by scratching or abrasion (Fig. 1.27).

Ulcer

An ulcer results from loss of substance on a cutaneous surface exposing the inner layers or

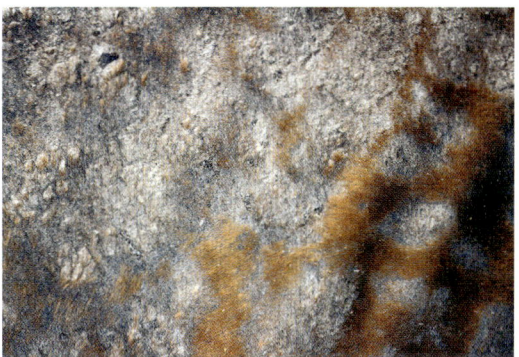

Fig. 1.23. Crusts and scaling in a horse diagnosed with sarcoidosis.

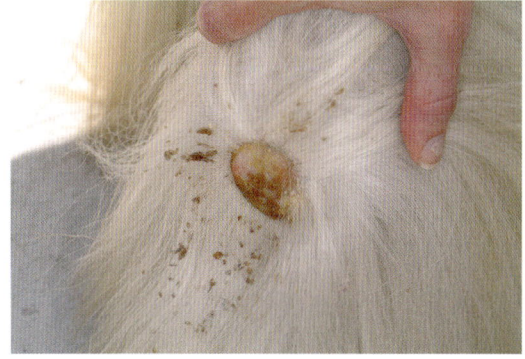

Fig. 1.24. Scaling due to the drying up of pustules in a horse diagnosed with *Chorioptes* infection.

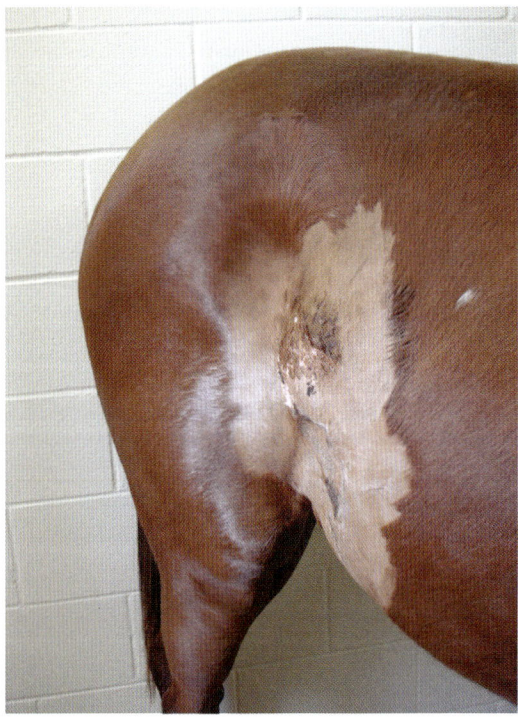

Fig. 1.25. Scar in a horse recovering from *Corynebacterium* infection.

tissues. There may be full-thickness loss of the epidermis. It can be the result of severe pruritus (Fig. 1.28) or the opening of a deeper lesion (Fig. 1.29)

Lichenification

This involves thickening of the skin with exaggeration of normal markings. It consists of acanthosis (increased thickness of the epidermis), hyperkeratosis (increased thickness of the stratum corneum) and dermal thickening. This is an indication of chronic disease. It is frequently associated with hyperpigmentation (Fig. 1.30).

Hyperpigmentation

Hyperpigmentation is increased pigmentation of the skin. This can be associated with increased thickness of the skin or the result of increased melanin production, as occurs with tanning.

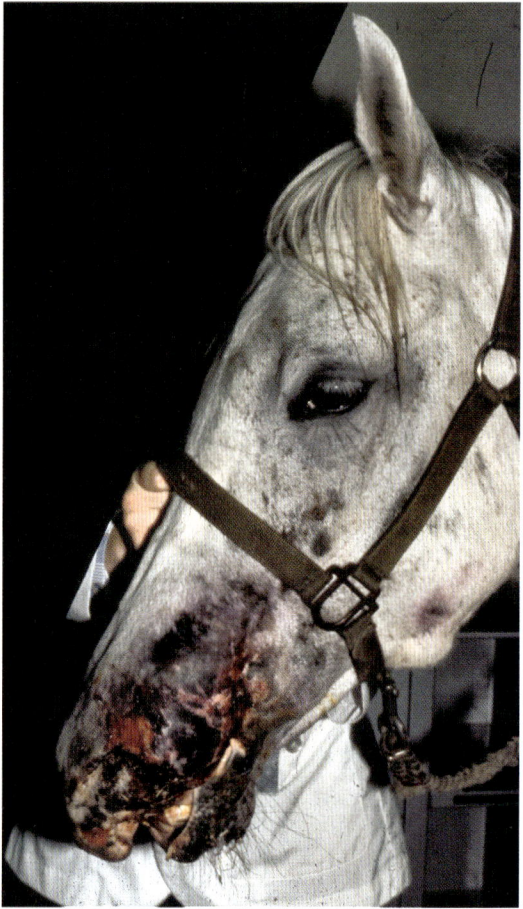

Fig. 1.26. Severe scarring in a horse with pythiosis and undergoing multiple surgical resections.

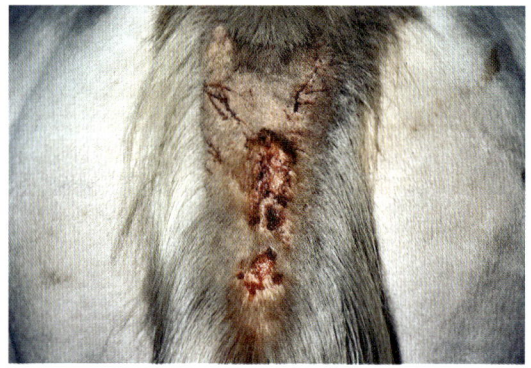

Fig. 1.27. Excoriations and ulcerations in a horse with uncontrolled insect allergies and extreme pruritus. The alopecia is the result of self-trauma.

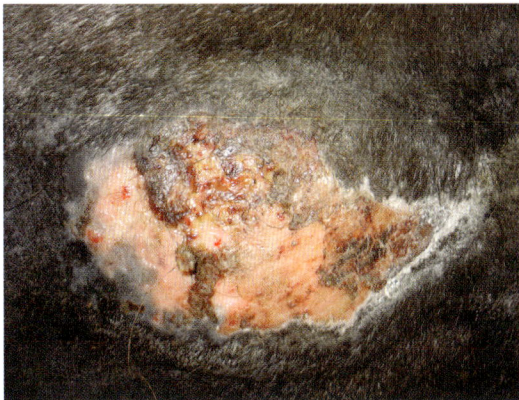

Fig. 1.28. Deep ulcerative lesions in a severe case of habronemiasis complicated by bacterial infection. Severe pruritus was present in this case.

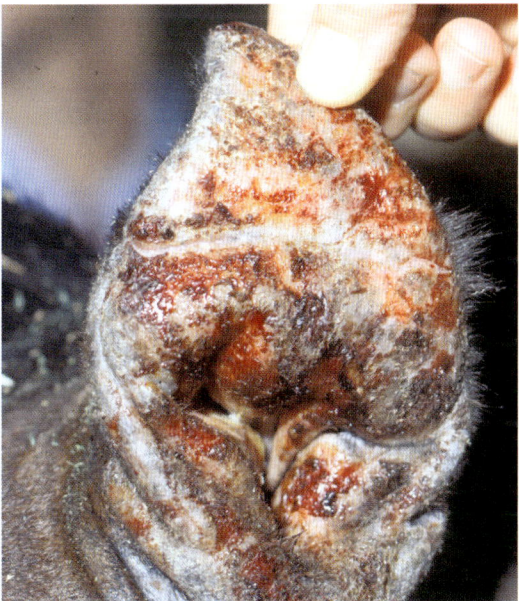

Fig. 1.29. Severe ulcerative lesions in a horse with *Culicoides* hypersensitivity, uncontrolled pruritus and secondary *Pseudomonas* infection.

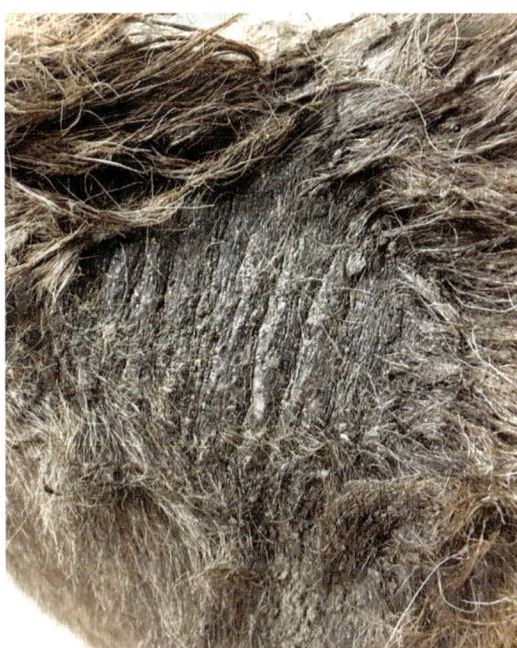

Fig. 1.30. Lichenification and hyperpigmentation in a horse with chronic skin disease.

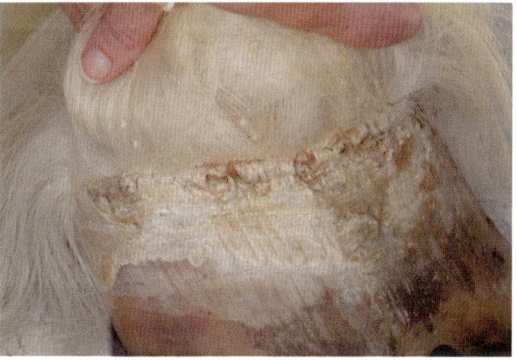

Fig. 1.31. Hyperkeratosis on the coronary band of a horse diagnosed with coronary band dystrophy.

Hyperkeratosis

Hyperkeratosis is thickening of the stratum corneum due to an increased number of keratinized cells (Fig. 1.31). It may result from increased production or decreased loss of cells. Orthokeratosis is a form of hyperkeratosis where the nucleus is lost in the normal fashion (compared with parakeratosis, where the nucleus is retained).

Differential diagnoses

After identification of the type of lesion and their distribution, the clinician can formulate a list of differential diagnoses and consider appropriate diagnostics to rule diseases in or out. Some tests are specific to dermatology (see Chapter 2, this volume), while others are general, such as blood tests.

Examples of common differential diagnoses for papular/pustular eruptions are:

- Allergic disease (e.g. *Culicoides* infection, contact, food);
- Mites (e.g. *Chorioptes* infection);
- Folliculitis (bacterial and fungal infections);
- Immune-mediated disease (less common), e.g. pemphigus.

Differential diagnoses for nodules/plaques include:

- Infectious disease (e.g. bacterial, fungal, viral);
- Allergic disease (e.g. eosinophilic granuloma);
- Immune-mediated disease (e.g. erythema multiforme);
- Neoplastic disease (e.g. sarcoid, melanoma).

2 Diagnostic Tests in Dermatology

Based on the differential diagnoses and their ranking, the clinician will decide which diseases to rule out first and which diagnostic tests are most helpful. It is important to note that some diseases are diagnosed by exclusion of others, while other diseases can be positively diagnosed with a specific test. For example, atopic dermatitis is a clinical diagnosis and there is no diagnostic test per se for this disease; thus, diagnosis of atopic dermatitis is based on clinical signs, a suggestive history, compatible clinical signs and exclusion of other pruritic diseases with similar symptoms. Allergy testing is not used for diagnostic purposes, only to identify allergens to include for immunotherapy. In contrast, in the case of dermatophytosis, diagnosis is based on a positive fungal culture.

Knowing which tests are most helpful and how to prioritize them is important. For example, if the clinician suspects both contact allergy and food allergy, it is important to know that contact allergy can be ruled out more quickly than food allergy. Indeed, contact allergy can be diagnosed after 7–10 days of confinement, while food allergy may require 2 months of food trials. For these diseases, blood work is not helpful in making a diagnosis.

This chapter describes the most common diagnostic tests carried out in dermatology with a brief description of how to perform them.

Skin Scraping

Skin scraping is cheap, easy to perform and often remarkably informative. It should be performed in most dermatoses as part of the minimum work-up. Hair should be clipped from the sites that are going to be scraped. A dull, clean #10 scalpel blade should be used. Some dermatologists instead use a small metal spatula. Good-quality, heavy-grade mineral oil is placed directly on to the skin and the slide. If a mite infection is suggested in the differential diagnosis, the scraping may be superficial or deep, depending on the habits of the mite being

considered. For example, *Chorioptes* spp. are superficial mites and therefore large, superficial scrapings are ideal for their detection. The preferred body sites for this mite are the lower legs and the coronary band area.

For deep scrapings, pinch or squeeze the skin, scrape until you get capillary oozing and then pinch, scrape, pinch again and scrape again. Plucking hairs can also be a useful adjunct to deep skin scraping for areas that are difficult to scrape. Place the debris in the mineral oil and distribute it evenly. Add a coverslip to decrease the depth of field and protect your microscope. This is very important to ensure that all the material is more or less in the same plane of vision. Use low lighting (e.g. close the condenser) and 100× magnification. The low light is important as bright light may greatly decrease the ability to see the mites.

Direct Examination of Hair and Scales

Hair shaft morphology

Direct examination of hairs can provide useful information, although it may not be a very sensitive approach for the diagnosis of dermatophytes or other abnormalities. This is because some diseases are focal and not all areas are affected equally. It is also a time-consuming test to do in multiple areas. Ten to 20 hairs can be plucked by pulling in the same direction of the hair growth to increase the likelihood of getting the whole hair and not breaking the root. Hairs are positioned in an orderly array on the slide and a drop of mineral oil is added to increase adherence of the hairs to the slide. The use of a coverslip is important to facilitate flattening and examination of the hairs in the same plane. Hairs can be examined for broken ends, frayed cuticles and melanin clumping. It is important to note whether the hairs are in the telogen or anagen phase and to examine for deformity of the hair or of the bulb in cases of alopecia areata or dysplasia. In healthy individuals, the majority of hairs from the body in horses are in the telogen phase, while those on the mane and tail are in anagen phase.

Examination for superficial fungi

Dermatophytes can be seen on direct examination of the hair, although this is not a sensitive method for diagnosis. If present, the dermatophyte is present as arthrospores on the cortex of the hair shaft. An agent that will clear keratin is useful for examination. Three that are used for this purpose are: (i) 10–20% potassium hydroxide (KOH); (ii) KOH + dimethyl sulfoxide (DMSO); and (iii) chlorphenolac. In heavily infected hairs, it is possible to see spores in mineral oil preparations. However, this is not a very sensitive test and therefore negative findings are not interpreted as an accurate way to rule out dermatophytosis. Importantly, even if positive findings are detected, a fungal culture should always be done to positively identify which dermatophyte is responsible for the infection.

After an appropriate amount of clearing time, the hairs can be examined for signs of fungal-induced damage. Use 400× magnification on damaged hairs to inspect for the presence of arthrospores. This is not an easy diagnostic test to master and it is not done by most practitioners.

Cytology

Cytology is by far the most common test done in equine dermatology.

Surface cytology

Surface cytology is done using Scotch tape. It is fast and inexpensive, and can provide much useful information. Tape can be placed on areas of alopecia and scaling to collect keratinocytes and identify the cells in the crusts. Tape cytology is not easy to read and requires some expertise as there is frequently a lot of material on the slide. It is important to scan the slide to identify the most helpful areas, such as areas where there are leukocytes. Identification of intracellular bacteria is ideal to make a diagnosis of bacterial infection, although *Staphylococcus* spp. are often seen extracellularly. The clinicians will have to use their judgement when interpreting the results of cytology as there is no magic number for bacteria or yeast to define it as an infection that warrants treatment. Tape cytology is commonly done, as pustules are transient and rarely found

intact. If pustules are present, they are a much better area to sample.

Impression smears/aspirations

Impression smears from moist lesions or pustules are often very useful to provide information regarding the type of exudate and the presence of organisms. Nodules, intact pustules and vesicles can be aspirated with 22–25G needles. The cells are aspirated into the needle and can then be blown on to the slide with air from the syringe and smeared into a monolayer. Pustules are the ideal lesion to examine for acantholytic cells. Exudative lesions can be touched, swabbed or lightly scraped to produce thin smears on a clean slide. Copious exudate can be mounted in a drop of KOH or in a wet stain such as new methylene blue. Except for wet preparations, slides should be air dried. For impression smears of skin and ear swabs, heat fixation is usually advocated. Sometimes, only thick crusts are available. This may be the case in chronic cases of dermatophilosis or pemphigus foliaceus. Sometimes, it is useful to cut the crust into small pieces and add some saline to moisten the preparation.

Diff-Quik is the most common stain for cytology at the time of visit. Special stains can be used on skin biopsies to visualize specific organisms. For example, acid-fast stains such as Ziehl–Neelsen or Fite Faraco can be used if *Nocardia* or *Mycobacterium* spp. are suspected, while PAS (periodic acid–Schiff) or GMS (Grocott-Gomori's or Gömöri methenamine silver stain) can be used for fungi.

Dermatophyte Culture

Although dermatophytes are not common in immunocompetent horses, fungal cultures are a common part of the dermatological work-up and are critical in cases of crusting and patchy hair loss in young or elderly horses. Cultures for dermatophytes are done by collecting hairs in small numbers from the edge of an affected lesion. New lesions that are increasing in size are the best areas to sample as the dermatophyte expands peripherally. Usually, the hairs are prepped with alcohol and allowed to dry. This helps to decrease the number of contaminant saprophytes. The hairs are gently laid on Sabouraud medium and kept at room temperature. Preparation of the skin is crucial in horses due to the heavy presence of saprophytes on their skin.

As some equine dermatophytes require vitamin B to grow, it is important to add a drop of vitamin B complex to the plate to encourage the growth of these organisms and prevent a false-negative result. More specifically, *Trichophyton verrucosum* requires thiamine and inositol. One approach to provide both ingredients is to add yeast extract to the Sabouraud agar, as the extract is rich in both inositol and thiamine. Failure to do this may lead to a negative culture. *Trichophyton equinum* requires niacin to grow. Once again, adding a few drops of vitamin B complex ensures that this essential vitamin is available to the dermatophyte.

Dermatophyte test medium (DTM) is essentially Sabouraud dextrose agar containing antibacterial and antifungal agents plus a color indicator (phenol red). This is because dermatophytes utilize the protein first in the medium and the alkaline metabolites change the color of the plate from yellow to red. Other fungi use carbohydrates first and then proteins. For this reason, it is important to evaluate the plate daily in the first 10 days. After the first 2 weeks, other fungi will turn the medium red and this should not be interpreted as a positive dermatophyte culture result.

It is important to note that Wood's lamp examination is not typically done in equine dermatology, unless it is being done to identify *Microsporum canis*. Approximately 50% of *M. canis* will fluoresce using this procedure. *M. canis* is a rare cause of dermatophytosis in horses. The other dermatophytes affecting horses (e.g. *T. equinum*) do not fluoresce, so Wood's lamp examination is of limited value in equine dermatology.

Biopsy

When the lesion is confined to the upper dermis and epidermis, lidocaine can be introduced with a fine needle subcutaneously just below the biopsy site. For deeper lesions, general anesthesia may be required.

No surgical preparation should be performed other than atraumatic clipping for samples that are submitted for dermatopathology. This is crucial, as prepping will remove the scales and crusts and damage fragile lesions that may be necessary to obtain a diagnosis. This is different in the case of samples that are biopsied to be submitted for culture. In these cases, the surface of the skin is surgically prepared to increase the likelihood of culturing the primary deep pathogen in the skin.

Small superficial lesions (less than 2–4 mm) can be biopsied with disposable biopsy punches. Punches of 4 and 6 mm are the most useful. Larger lesions may need to be excised. In the case of nodular dermatitis, it is most helpful to remove an unerupted intact nodule if possible and to submit it for both histopathology and culture.

The most important step in the biopsy procedure is selecting a primary lesion. Biopsy of secondary skin changes is often unrewarding. The second most important step is finding a pathologist with some expertise in veterinary dermatology.

Intradermal Skin Test

An intradermal skin test (also called an intradermal test or skin test) is not diagnostic for allergies, as positive results can be seen in horses that are pruritic for reasons other than allergies, or even in normal horses. The purpose of an intradermal skin test is to detect the allergens to which the horse has developed allergen-specific IgE detectable in the skin. Intradermal skin testing should only be considered once a clinical diagnosis of allergy has been made and the clinician is attempting to identify suitable allergens for the formulation of allergen-specific immunotherapy.

With intradermal testing, very small amounts of a very dilute preparation of antigens are injected intradermally (0.05 ml containing 1000 PNU (protein nitrogen units) for most antigens). In horses, the response to the injected antigen is read 15–30 min after injection (Fig. 2.1). The responses are compared with negative and positive controls and subjectively graded from 0 to 4, where 0 is the score given to the reaction to saline (negative control) and 4+ is the score of the histamine reaction (positive control; given as histamine phosphate diluted 1:100,000). Scores of 2 or higher are considered positive reactions.

All results must be analyzed in light of the patient's history and signs. Drugs and stress can interfere with a positive skin test, and therefore it is recommended to discontinue glucocorticoids and antihistamines prior to the test. The withdrawal time depends on the horse, dose and duration of therapy. Few studies have been done on this topic; one published study evaluated skin test reactivity in horses without signs of atopic dermatitis but only evaluated the effects of dexamethasone and hydroxyzine (Petersen and Schott, 2009). Each drug was only given for 1 week, which is not how these

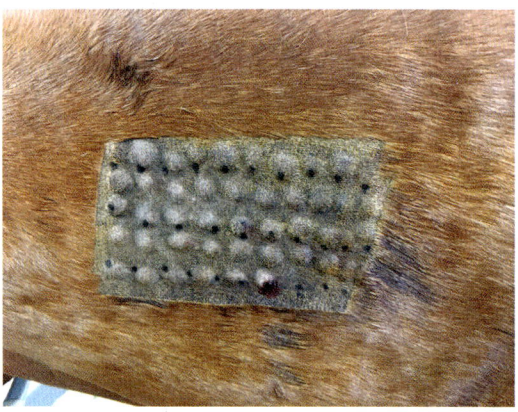

Fig. 2.1. Intradermal skin test in an allergic horse. The first injection (top left corner) is saline, which is the negative control. The second injection is histamine (the positive control, scored as 4+). All other injections (tested allergens) are scored for size, firmness and erythema by comparing them with the two controls. Some examples of strong positives in this horse are the fifth injection on the top row and the first injections on the second and third rows.

medications are prescribed in real life. The authors concluded that a withdrawal of 1 week for antihistamines and 2 weeks for dexamethasone is recommended prior to intradermal testing. These times are those that general clinicians use as a reference, although it is important to remember that variability exists among horses, and some horses can have a very good skin test even with shorter withdrawal times.

It is important to remember that a positive response does not render a diagnosis of allergy as antibodies can be seen in asymptomatic horses; thus, the significance and relevance of the clinical signs observed come from the overall assessment of the clinician.

Another approach to identify allergens to which the horse has built up an IgE response is a serology test. This approach will be discussed in more depth in Chapter 5 (this volume). Briefly, it has been demonstrated that a serology test is not useful for the diagnosis of food allergy and needs to be interpreted carefully in the context of environmental allergies because positive tests can be found in non-symptomatic horses or in horses that are pruritic for other reasons. Variations also exist depending on the methodology and the company selected to carry out the serology test, and therefore care should be taken to select a reputable company with good-quality controls that can provide repeatable results. Serology does not typically correlate with the results of intradermal skin testing for a variety of reasons. It is also commonly accepted that drugs have less ability to interfere with a serology test and therefore discontinuation of medications is less critical and is not frequently recommended prior to serology testing.

Patch Test

A patch test can be done to investigate the possibility of contact allergy. In this case, samples of suspected allergens (e.g. shavings, plants, topical products used on the animal) are applied to small patches and the patches are placed on a shaved area (typically on the lateral neck) (Figs 2.2–2.5). The patches are left in place for 24 h. After this period of time, the patches are removed and the skin is examined for the presence of papules or vesicles, which are indicative of a positive response. However, a positive response on an allergy test does not necessarily mean that this is the cause of the problem. The results need to be interpreted taking into account the history and clinical signs.

Culture

Culture is frequently indicated in veterinary dermatology. Routine bacterial culture and sensitivity testing are done increasingly frequently in bacterial pyodermas, as *Staphylococcus* spp. are becoming resistant to antibiotics. For superficial pyodermas, the ideal lesion to culture is a pustule. If pustules are present, rupture of an intact pustule is recommended with no aseptic preparation. A drop of pus should be collected on a culturette. For deep pyoderma, it is important to clean an intact lesion and then express pus on the culturette. An even better approach is to biopsy a nodule that has not opened and drained yet, and to remove the whole nodule and submit it for culture. In this case, the surface of the skin is surgically prepared to remove superficial contaminants so that only the deep pathogen is cultured. The biopsy sample should be kept cool and moist during transport to the laboratory in a sterile container. Deep nodules are typically cultured for bacteria (aerobic and anaerobic), atypical mycobacteria and fungi.

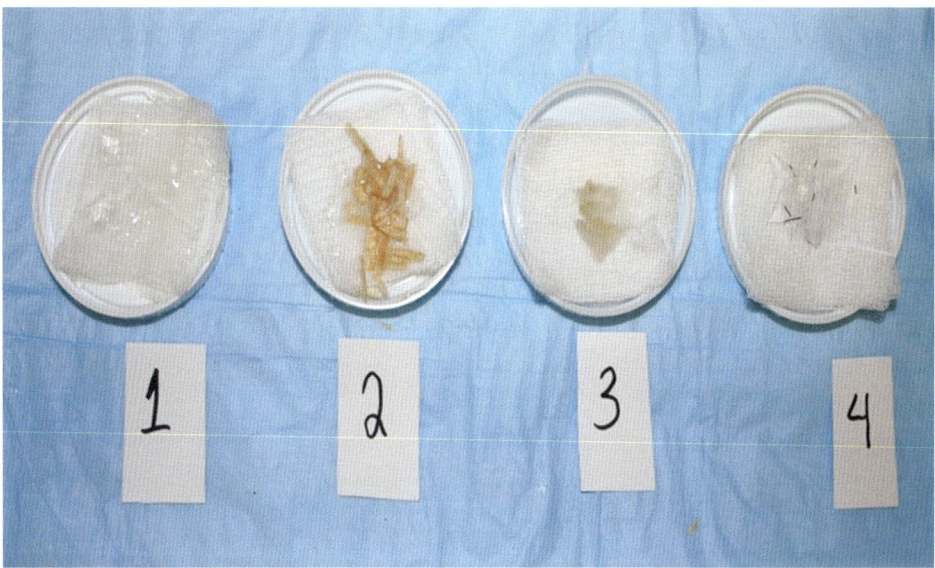

Fig. 2.2. Examples of allergens used for patch testing. 1, control (Vaseline); 2, pine shavings; 3, fleece from the horse's blanket; 4, a small amount of shampoo used on the horse.

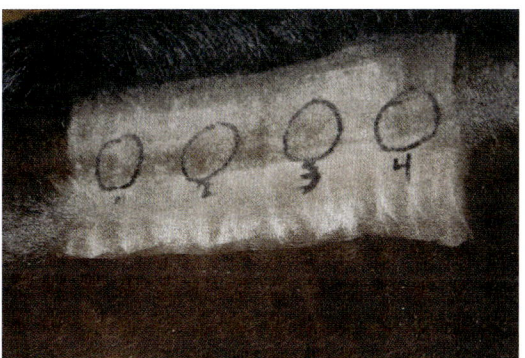
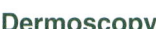

Fig. 2.3. Once prepared, the patches described in Fig. 2.2 are placed on a shaved area of the neck.

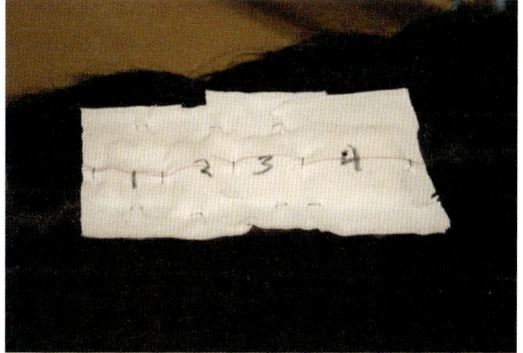

Fig. 2.4. The patches described in Fig. 2.2 are then secured on the side of the neck. In this case, soft bandages were chosen to keep the patches in place. Mane tamers are another option.

Dermoscopy

Dermoscopy is a diagnostic tool used in human medicine and in small animals for evaluation of the hair and skin surface. It is a non-invasive imaging technique typically used for evaluation of pigmented lesions. Although this technique is not routinely done in equine practice, it could become another useful tool in equine dermatology. Recently, a study in horses demonstrated its feasibility and ease of use (Legnani *et al.*, 2018). Although this study only assessed feasibility, it is possible to speculate that this technique may be an alternative to differentiate occult sarcoids from dermatophytes or other infections, thereby avoiding the need and potential risk of worsening of the sarcoid by performing a biopsy.

Important Take-home Message

Of all the diagnostic tests available in dermatology, the most commonly used are cytology, skin scraping

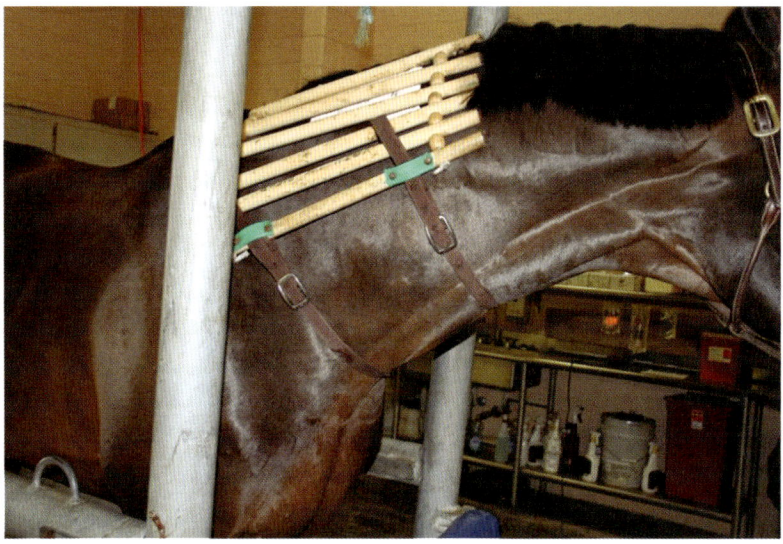

Fig. 2.5. A rigid device may be used instead of soft bandages or mane tamers to protect the patch test area.

and biopsy. Careful interpretation of the results is important to make the most of these tests. Cytology requires some experience and practice in identifying the most informative areas on the slide, particularly when doing tape cytology. When biopsy is chosen, it is crucial not to scrub the area, and to select a primary lesion if at all possible. Secondary lesions, open nodules and ulcerated areas are of limited usefulness and should not be selected for biopsy. If allergy testing is pursued, it is important to remember that it has no diagnostic value for allergy; instead, the results should be interpreted in the context of the clinical history and presentation to aid in the selection of allergens to avoid or to include for allergen-specific immunotherapy.

References

Legnani, S., Zini, E., Roccabianca, P., Funiciello, B. and Zanna, G. (2018) Dermoscopic analysis of the skin of healthy warmblood horses: a descriptive study of 34 cases in Italy. *Veterinary Dermatology* 29, 165-e61.

Petersen, A. and Schott, H.C. (2009) Effects of dexamethasone and hydroxyzine treatment on intradermal testing and allergen-specific IgE serum testing results in horses. *Veterinary Dermatology* 20, 615–622.

Further Reading

Dupont, S., de Spiegeleer, A., Liu, D.J.X., Lefère, L., van Doorn, D.A. and Hesta, M. (2016) A commercially available immunoglobulin E-based test for food allergy gives inconsistent results in healthy ponies. *Equine Veterinary Journal* 48, 109–113.

Jose-Cunilleras, E., Kohn, C.W., Hillier, A., Saville, W.J.A. and Lorch, G. (2001) Intradermal testing in healthy horses and horses with chronic obstructive pulmonary disease, recurrent urticaria, or allergic dermatitis. *Journal of the American Veterinary Medical Association* 219, 1115–1121.

Lebis, C., Bourdeau, P. and Marzin-Keller, F. (2002) Intradermal skin tests in equine dermatology: a study of 83 horses. *Equine Veterinary Journal* 34, 666–671.

3 Dermatological Therapy

Dermatological therapy is frequently a combination of systemic medications with topical therapy. In milder cases, topical therapy may be the only therapy. It is important for clinicians to know whether systemic therapy is necessary or not. For example, indiscriminate use of a systemic antibiotic can be contraindicated. At the same time, it is important to understand when infections are deep enough and chronic enough that application of a topical antibiotic will not be sufficient to resolve the problem.

Topical Therapy: General Principles

Topical therapy is an essential component in the treatment of many dermatological diseases, whether alone or in conjunction with systemic therapy. Topical therapy has many advantages, such as delivering a high concentration of medication directly on to the target organ and thus minimizing the risk of adverse effects. This is the case for drugs such as glucocorticoids. It also has the potential to correct skin barrier defects by delivering lipid compounds that may be deficient in some patients. As our knowledge of skin barrier impairment increases, the opportunity to explore skin barrier repair topically is highly appealing and promising. Topical therapy is also beneficial to decrease the penetration of allergens in allergic patients and to provide immediate relief of pruritus through the use of cool water and soothing ingredients. Importantly, topical therapy can minimize the need for systemic antimicrobial therapy, which is of immense benefit, as antibacterial resistance is becoming increasingly common. Many of the shampoos used for horses are small-animal products that also have a label for horses, and only a few products have been specifically developed and marketed for horses. As a general rule, areas with long, thick hairs (e.g. the pastern in feathered horses) may need to be clipped to increase the efficacy of topical therapy. A shorter coat allows the use of less product and allows direct contact with the affected area. As a basic principle, dry skin can be itchy and needs to be moisturized, while moist lesions should be dried and therefore occlusive treatment using ointments and creams would be contraindicated. Contact time is essential for the success of topical therapy when using shampoos or conditioners that are not designed to be left on. If the product is rinsed away too quickly, it may not have had sufficient time to exert its effect. For this reason, most dermatologists suggest a 5–10 min contact time before rinsing.

Topical Therapy in the Allergic Patient

Currently, we understand that the epicutaneous route of allergen penetration is extremely important in atopic dermatitis in humans and dogs. We do not know if this also applies to allergy in horses, but it is reasonable to speculate that it may also be the case in this species. Allergic individuals typically have some form of skin barrier defect, either primary or secondary due to inflammation and self-trauma. Application of allergens to a defective barrier promotes a T-helper type 2 cell response and allergic sensitization. Thus, allergic patients need topical therapy at many different levels. The most immediate reason is that shampoo therapy removes allergens and minimizes the time that such allergens stay on the skin. This is why it is desirable for owners to bathe allergic horses frequently using mild hypoallergenic shampoos. Cool water provides relief from itching and temporarily moisturizes the skin. The second reason for topical therapy in allergic patients is to decrease pruritus and inflammation and to minimize the use of systemic glucocorticoids. In acute flares, the use of topical glucocorticoids can calm down inflammation rapidly and minimize the development of a secondary infection and self-trauma. Skin care with soothing agents is helpful to decrease pruritus. Many owners of allergic horses comment on the fact that the horse seems more comfortable and less pruritic after bathing with moisturizing, soothing ingredients such as oatmeal, ceramides, fatty acids and pramoxine to decrease the itch.

It is also known that proactive therapy twice a week with topical glucocorticoids in areas where the patient is prone to develop dermatitis is beneficial to reduce the frequency and severity of flares. This strategy is known as "proactive therapy" as opposed to "reactive therapy," which takes place once the lesions have already occurred. The value of this approach is well documented in human medicine but has only recently been introduced in veterinary medicine. For this reason, spraying an allergic horse with a spray containing some hydrocortisone twice a week can be an effective way to prevent major flares while minimizing the need for rescue medications during the worst part of the allergy season.

In the long term, allergic patients also benefit from topical therapy aimed at restoration of the skin barrier. Alterations of the ultrastructure of the epidermis have been demonstrated in allergic horses compared with normal horses. Although we do not know yet what alterations are present in the skin lipids of allergic horses, we know that the serum lipids of allergic horses are different from those of healthy controls and that these changes correlate with their clinical status and the severity of their allergies. In particular, allergic horses have less phosphatidylcholine and sphingomyelin compared with healthy controls, and sphingomyelin is specifically correlated with the clinical status.

A positive response to ceramide deficiency in atopic dermatitis in other species has been seen with both topical therapy using sphingolipid emulsions and oral supplementation with essential fatty acids. Although no study has been done to document ceramide deficiency in the skin of allergic horses, ceramide-based shampoos and sprays are also available for horses and are frequently prescribed to soothe the irritated skin of allergic horses, with a good response in clinics.

The most common antipruritic ingredients in topical therapy include oatmeal, topical anesthetics such as pramoxine, some form of emollient or moisturizer, and a topical glucocorticoid such as hydrocortisone. When more powerful relief is needed, some clinicians add injectable dexamethasone to either fly sprays or antimicrobial commercially available sprays. The amount of dexamethasone added is calculated to provide a final concentration of 0.01%. The stability of these preparations is unknown when dexamethasone is added in this

way and therefore they need to be used within a few days. Another more expensive option is the use of human products that include more powerful fluorinated steroids. This is typically done only for small areas and is not feasible for use on the whole body. It is important to note that chronic use of topical glucocorticoids, particularly if under occlusion, can lead to cutaneous atrophy and poor healing. Therefore, this needs to be done carefully and with monitoring.

Another powerful antipruritic agent is lime sulfur. This product is used in veterinary dermatology for a variety of reasons and its antipruritic effect is one of them. It also has keratolytic, antifungal and antiparasitic properties.

Topical Antimicrobial Therapy for Bacteria and Yeasts

Many dermatology patients are prone to frequent secondary infections. Topical antimicrobial therapy is an essential adjunctive treatment for the management of pyoderma. Residual antimicrobial activity is highly variable depending on the formulation of the product selected, and thus it is important to note that not all antimicrobials perform similarly. It should also be noted that topical therapy with chlorhexidine digluconate products can be as effective as systemic therapy, at least in other species. Very few controlled studies have been done in horses, but one published study showed that topical therapy with stannous fluoride was an effective treatment for pyoderma, minimizing the need for systemic antibiotics (Marsella and Akucewich, 2007). This is very important, as antibiotic resistance is becoming more prevalent in all species, including horses. The efficacy of a shampoo is dependent not only on the concentration of the active ingredients but also on the shampoo formulation. For example, in one study, dog hair shafts treated with shampoos containing 2% or 3% chlorhexidine and the combination of shampoo and conditioner showed significantly inhibited bacterial growth, indicating that this is a suitable treatment for bacterial pyoderma (Kloos et al., 2013).

Horses with staphylococcal pyoderma benefit from topical therapy with either chlorhexidine or benzoyl peroxide. It is important to remember that benzoyl peroxide has an overall higher drying ability than chlorhexidine. It removes crusts and helps with follicular flushing. While it can be beneficial initially when the horse has many crusts, it may dry the skin too much if used too frequently or for extended periods of time. In such cases, the dry skin can be pruritic so this can be counterproductive. The use of moisturizing conditions or switching to a milder and more soothing preparation may be needed. Triclosan is another effective antimicrobial ingredient present in some veterinary products that can be used for equine pyoderma. Wipes containing chlorhexidine, climbazole and Tris-EDTA buffer can also be used for localized infections, particularly on the face, which would be difficult to shampoo. This type of product would be helpful against both bacteria and yeasts.

Iodine is typically not an effective strategy for the treatment of pyoderma in horses and frequently causes irritation. Therefore, it is not routinely recommended in dermatological patients.

Products containing oxychlorine are frequently used for spot treatment of bacterial infections. They are typically well tolerated and effective but require frequent use (two to three times a day) and are rather expensive if used on large areas of the body.

Topical Therapy for Dermatophytosis

Dermatophytosis is typically a self-limiting disease in horses, and topical therapy is frequently used as the only treatment for dermatophytosis in horses. In a randomized clinical trial, a mixture of tea tree oil and enilconazole rinses was found to be an effective protocol (Pisseri et al., 2009). Enilconazole wash or spray and natamycin spray are the primary topical options used in many European countries. Enilconazole is typically used at intervals of 3–4 days for a maximum of four times. Other protocols call for repeated body rinses with an enilconazole solution or miconazole with or without chlorhexidine.

In the USA, lime sulfur is the most commonly prescribed topical treatment for whole-body treatment of dermatophytosis in horses. It is commonly prescribed once a week for 4–5 weeks. It will temporarily stain the coat yellow, and owners of white horses need to be aware of this adverse effect to avoid surprises. Lime sulfur has also an offensive sulfur smell. It is highly antipruritic and keratolytic, and is useful against mites.

Topical Therapy for Parasites

The most common mite that is treated in horses is *Chorioptes* spp. This mange is particularly common in feathered horses. As it is a superficial mite, systemic therapy frequently fails to resolve the infestation and the single most important therapy is topical therapy. In order to increase the efficacy of this therapy and ensure good contact of the product with the skin, it is best to clip the area. The efficacy of treatment is also increased if, prior to application of the insecticide, the area is shampooed with a keratolytic/antimicrobial agent such as benzoyl peroxide to help remove some of the crusts and kill bacteria. To kill the mites, lime sulfur dips (once a week for 4–5 weeks) are frequently prescribed in the USA. It is important to make sure that the animal does not get wet in between dips to maintain sufficient residual activity.

Another effective option is topical eprinomectin, which is useful for both *Chorioptes* and *Psoroptes* mites. The life cycle of the mites is approximately 3 weeks, and therefore the treatment needs to be extended to cover and exceed the life cycle by 1 week. Importantly, *Chorioptes* mites can survive off the host for several months and therefore environmental application of insecticides such as pyrethrins may be needed to avoid reinfestation.

Systemic Therapies for Pruritus

Unfortunately, limited options are available to relieve pruritus in horses. In small-animal dermatology, multiple options besides glucocorticoids are available to decrease allergic pruritus systemically; in contrast, very few are available in horses. This is because little is known regarding the mediators of itch in horses.

Relief of pruritus in horses is dependent largely on the use of glucocorticoids, either topically or systemically. Other treatments used in dogs, such as Janus kinase (JAK) inhibitors or biologics, are not currently available in horses. Antihistamines have limited efficacy for relief of pruritus in horses, probably because histamine is not a main mediator of pruritus in this species. This is confirmed by the observation that urticaria (hives) is not a pruritic disease in horses, although it is in other species. A study using cetirizine to relieve pruritus in insect-allergic horses failed to report any benefit (Olsén et al., 2011). The lack of major benefit with the use of antihistamines for pruritus is typically the experience in the field, regardless of the antihistamine used. Thus, antihistamines are used primarily for hives in horses but not usually as monotherapy for pruritus in allergic horses, although some practitioners still use them. As is the case in other species, the response to antihistamines is highly variable among individuals, and different antihistamines may need to be tried to find the most suitable one for each case. Frequently considered antihistamines are hydroxyzine (0.5–1 mg/kg of body weight every 8 h), chlorpheniramine (0.25 mg/kg every 12 h) and diphenhydramine (1 mg/kg every 12 h).

Glucocorticoids are used for both allergic and immune-mediated diseases in horses. The two most commonly prescribed glucocorticoids in equine practice are prednisolone and dexamethasone. It is important to use prednisolone rather than prednisone in horses to avoid treatment failure, as horses do not metabolize prednisone to prednisolone. Oral prednisolone is considered the safest approach, with a very low risk for laminitis unless the horse has a previous history of it or another predisposing disease such as metabolic syndrome. Regardless of the choice, these drugs are typically prescribed initially daily, for an induction period, which can range from 7 to 14 days, followed by tapering and alternate-day regimens over a period of several weeks. Every attempt should be made to find the lowest effective dose and the least frequent administration necessary to control the disease. For prednisolone, the induction dose used for allergic diseases is typically 0.5–1.5 mg/kg/day and the maintenance dose is 0.2–0.5 mg/kg every other day or less. For autoimmune diseases, the induction dose for prednisolone is typically 1.5–2.5 mg/kg/day and the maintenance dose is 0.5–1 mg/kg every other day or less. If prednisolone is not effective, dexamethasone can be tried. A common loading dose is 0.05–0.1 mg/kg, followed by 0.01–0.02 mg/kg every 48–72 h. Monitoring for laminitis and other adverse effects is essential with long-term use of glucocorticoids.

Oral supplementation with flaxseed has been reported to be somewhat helpful for horses allergic to *Culicoides* spp. midges. In one study, allergic horses were randomized to receive either 200 ml of linseed oil (*n*-3 source) or 200 ml of maize oil (*n*-6 source) per day for a 6-week period (Friberg and Logas, 1999). After a 6-week washout period, each horse was crossed over to the other supplement for an additional 6 weeks. Horses were evaluated every 3 weeks. Although there was no significant change in the level of pruritus observed between the groups, most owners stated that horses improved while being supplemented with linseed oil. For this reason, this type of supplementation can be considered as a helpful adjunctive treatment in allergic horses as it is well tolerated and may decrease the dependence on glucocorticoids.

Recently, a new approach has been considered to decrease signs of allergic skin disease. While an actual biologic is not available for horses, a study was published using a vaccine against interleukin (IL)-5 in *Culicoides*-hypersensitive horses (Fettelschoss-Gabriel *et al.*, 2018). IL-5 was selected due to the fact that it is an important cytokine in eosinophilic inflammation, although no prior studies had specifically shown that this is a key mediator of insect allergies in horses. In this study, 34 Icelandic horses were immunized with either placebo or IL-5. Clinical improvement by disease scoring showed that 47% and 21% of vaccinated horses reached 50% and 75% improvement, respectively. In the placebo group, no horse reached 75% improvement, and only 13% reached 50% improvement. The strategy to vaccinate an animal against its own cytokines currently seems like a drastic and potentially risky approach, as cytokines have multiple functions, many of which are linked to important immune functions. Additionally, while administering monoclonal antibodies is a short-lived strategy and requires repetitive injections to be sustained, the concept of vaccination can be potentially long lasting and less controllable in the event that adverse effects develop. Although this strategy could be the way of the future, it is important that large safety studies are done to investigate the unintended long-term consequences of this approach before introducing this therapy in the field.

Steroid-sparing Agents for Immune-mediated Diseases

Pentoxifylline is commonly prescribed in equine dermatology for allergic and immune-mediated diseases. This is especially the case for vasculitis. Pentoxifylline is a xanthine derivative related to caffeine and theophylline. It is a phosphodiesterase inhibitor and has a wide range of anti-inflammatory properties, as well as increasing blood flow and tissue oxygenation, all properties that can be beneficial in horses with vasculitis in the lower extremities. The commonly recommended dose is 8–10 mg/kg twice daily. While most horses tolerate this drug very well, some may show increased nervousness and cutaneous flushing. Pentoxifylline can also benefit horses with recurrent airway obstruction. For these reasons, this drug may be beneficial in allergic horses, particularly if they have both cutaneous and systemic manifestations of disease. No study has specifically assessed the effect of pentoxifylline as a monotherapy to decrease pruritus in allergic horses, although it is commonly prescribed in practice as an adjunctive treatment in allergic horses to minimize the dependence on glucocorticoids. Because it is very safe, it is a suitable long-term option.

Another drug that is sometimes used in equine dermatology for autoimmune cases as a steroid-sparing agent is azathioprine. The bioavailability of oral azathioprine has been reported to be low (1–7%), but its efficacy is anecdotal. Nevertheless, it is sometimes prescribed in association with glucocorticoids to decrease the amount and frequency of glucocorticoid administration. When the pharmacokinetics of this drug was studied, a single dose of 3 mg/kg was given either orally or intravenously (White *et al.*, 2005). The optimal oral dose for safe long-term immunosuppression in horses is not known; anecdotally, clinicians prescribe 3 mg/kg orally every 48 h.

Systemic Antibiotics in Dermatology

Dermatology patients frequently develop secondary infections caused by *Staphylococcus aureus*. Every effort should be made to treat skin infections topically, if at all possible. This is for two reasons. First, frequent use of systemic antibiotics promotes antibiotic resistance. As infections in dermatology patients are often recurrent until the underlying cause is properly corrected (which can be a challenge in severely allergic patients), it is possible that multiple rounds of treatments may be needed, which is one of the reasons why so much antibiotic resistance is seen in dermatology. Second, skin infections require long periods of treatment due to the nature of the infection – most antibiotics do not reach the skin well, requiring doses higher than those used for infections in other organs, as well as longer treatment times. These factors place the patient at risk for adverse effects. Topical therapy has the advantage of delivering the product right where it is needed and has no systemic adverse effects. Some cases, however, are too severe to be treated topically and require systemic antibiotic therapy.

As the pathogen in superficial pyoderma is typically a *Staphylococcus* sp., antibiotics used in dermatology typically are those targeting this organism. As the course for superficial pyoderma lasts several weeks, oral sulfonamides are the drug of choice for the vast majority of superficial pyoderma cases. For Trimethoprim/Sulfamethoxazole doses of 15–25 mg/kg every 12–24 h are typically recommended. Colitis is a possible adverse effect, and therefore close monitoring for diarrhea or any evidence of colic is important. The author has found that administration of probiotics helps to minimize gastrointestinal distress and diarrhea in these cases. Sulfonamides are also very effective for *Dermatophilus* infection. Many horses with dermatophilosis will also have a secondary staphylococcal infection. Injectable penicillins are sometimes used, although the use of injectable drugs for a couple of weeks is not ideal.

Due to the development of multidrug resistance, it is sometimes necessary to use other antibiotics that are less than ideal. One option for resistant staphylococcal infections is rifampin. This antibiotic is able to penetrate granulation and scar tissue. Liver toxicity and rapid resistance are two of the major downsides of this antibiotic. Therefore, liver enzyme monitoring and combination with other antibiotics to decrease the development of resistance are usually carried out. Typically, a dose of 10 mg/kg once daily is used for skin infections.

Fluoroquinolones are sometimes prescribed for resistant skin infections. It is very important to minimize the use of fluoroquinolones unless it is necessary based on the results of a culture and on sensitivity. This is because the use of fluoroquinolones in other species has been demonstrated to promote antibiotic resistance. This category of drugs is concentration-dependent and therefore once-daily administration at a dose that is high enough above the mutation prevention concentration is important. Splitting the daily dose into two lower doses to be given twice daily is the wrong approach pharmacologically when dealing with fluoroquinolones, as each maximum serum concentration (C_{max}) value will be lower as it is dependent on the administered dose. It is better to have the total daily dose as one dose, once daily. However, it is important to note that very high doses of enrofloxacin can induce neurological and orthopedic adverse effects; therefore, a daily dose of 5 mg/kg is typically used in horses. Again, the use of broad-spectrum antibiotics should be limited to cases where it is necessary. Fluoroquinolones should not be used in young, growing horses.

Systemic Antifungals

As dermatophytosis in horses is typically a self-limiting disease, systemic therapy is rarely needed.

If it is needed, azoles could be considered. No pharmacokinetics studies of griseofulvin in horses have been published, and use of this medication is currently not recommended for the treatment of dermatophytosis.

Use of azoles is cost-prohibitive for most people. One study reported the pharmacokinetics of fluconazole in horses, showing that this medication has good oral bioavailability and could be a suitable option for fungal infections in horses (Latimer *et al.*, 2001). A loading dose of 14 mg/kg was followed by administration of 5 mg/kg every 24 h for 10 days. As fluconazole is highly water soluble and has a limited affinity for keratin and skin, residual activity in the skin is not prolonged.

Itraconazole is a better choice for skin, although it is expensive for use in horses. One study found that itraconazole administered as a solution had higher and more consistent absorption in horses than when administered as capsules (Davis *et al.*, 2005). The recommended dose is 5 mg/kg orally once daily.

The pharmacokinetics of oral terbinafine in horses has also been reported (Younkin *et al.*, 2017); however, due to adverse effects (although self-resolving), its use for dermatophytosis is not justified at this time.

Iodides (sodium and potassium iodide) remain the drug of choice for sporotrichosis in horses compared with itraconazole due to the lower cost. Potassium iodide can be given with food as a twice-daily suspension of 25 ml (concentration of 160 g in 400 ml). This category of drugs is typically well tolerated, although animals should be monitored for the development of iodism (e.g. lacrimation, naso-ocular discharge, scaling).

Conclusions and Take Home Messages

Topical therapy is an important component of the management of many dermatological conditions, either as monotherapy or as an adjunctive therapy to speed up recovery and minimize the use of systemic drugs. Although shampoo therapy can be time-consuming, it is beneficial for the physical removal of allergens such as pollen and dirt from the coat, as well as aiding in the application of a medicated product. Based on what is known in humans and dogs, skin barrier repair can be promoted using ceramide-based products. Many bacterial infections can be treated topically to minimize the use of systemic antibiotics and decrease the risk for antibiotic resistance. It is important to remember that the vehicles of topical products are just as important as the active ingredient

and that significant differences may exist among various commercial products. If systemic antibiotics are used, it is important to determine the pathogen and to understand how to use the antibiotic appropriately in terms of dose, frequency and duration of therapy to minimize failures and decrease the risk of relapses and the development of resistance.

Control of pruritus can be done topically or systemically. Systemically, the most effective treatment is still the use of glucocorticoids. Every effort should be made to control the underlying disease to minimize the dependence on glucocorticoids and to strive in the long run to use the lowest effective dose and to carry out alternate-day treatment whenever possible.

References

Davis, J.L., Salmon, J.H. and Papich, M.G. (2005) Pharmacokinetics and tissue distribution of itraconazole after oral and intravenous administration to horses. *American Journal of Veterinary Research* 66, 1694–1701.

Fettelschoss-Gabriel, A., Fettelschoss, V., Thoms, F., Giese, C., Daniel, M. *et al.* (2018) Treating insect-bite hypersensitivity in horses with active vaccination against IL-5. *Journal of Allergy and Clinical Immunology* 142, 1194–1205.e3.

Friberg, C.A. and Logas, D. (1999) Treatment of *Culicoides* hypersensitive horses with high-dose n-3 fatty acids: a double-blinded crossover study. *Veterinary Dermatology* 10, 117–122.

Kloos, I., Straubinger, R.K., Werckenthin, C. and Mueller, R.S. (2013) Residual antibacterial activity of dog hairs after therapy with antimicrobial shampoos. *Vet Dermatol* 24(2): 250–254.

Latimer, F.G., Colitz, C.M., Campbell, N.B. and Papich, M.G. (2001) Pharmacokinetics of fluconazole following intravenous and oral administration and body fluid concentrations of fluconazole following repeated oral dosing in horses. *American Journal of Veterinary Research* 62, 1606–1611.

Marsella, R. and Akucewich, L. (2007) Investigation on the clinical efficacy and tolerability of a 0.4% topical stannous fluoride preparation (MedEquine Gel) for the treatment of bacterial skin infections in horses: a prospective, randomized, double-blinded, placebo-controlled clinical trial. *Veterinary Dermatology* 18, 444–450.

Olsén, L., Bondesson, U., Broström, H., Olsson, U., Mazogi, B. *et al.* (2011) Pharmacokinetics and effects of cetirizine in horses with insect bite hypersensitivity. *Veterinary Journal* 187, 347–351.

Pisseri, F., Bertoli, A., Nardoni, S., Pinto, L., Pistelli, L. *et al.* (2009) Antifungal activity of tea tree oil from *Melaleuca alternifolia* against *Trichophyton equinum*: an *in vivo* assay. *Phytomedicine* 16, 1056–1058.

White, S.D., Maxwell, L.K., Szabo, N.J., Hawkins, J.L. and Kollias-Baker, C. (2005) Pharmacokinetics of azathioprine following single-dose intravenous and oral administration and effects of azathioprine following chronic oral administration in horses. *American Journal of Veterinary Research* 66, 1578–1583.

Younkin, T.J., Davis, E.G. and Kukanich, B. (2017) Pharmacokinetics of oral terbinafine in adult horses. *Journal of Veterinary Pharmacology and Therapeutics* 40, 342–347.

Further Reading

Topical therapy in the allergic patient

Hallamaa, R. and Batchu, K. (2016) Phospholipid analysis in sera of horses with allergic dermatitis and in matched healthy controls. *Lipids in Health and Disease* 15, 45–47.

Marsella, R., Johnson, C. and Ahrens, K. (2014) First case report of ultrastructural cutaneous abnormalities in equine atopic dermatitis. *Research in Veterinary Science* 97, 382–385.

Topical therapy for bacteria

Couto, N., Belas, A., Tilley, P., Couto, I., Gama, L.T. *et al.* (2013) Biocide and antimicrobial susceptibility of methicillin-resistant staphylococcal isolates from horses. *Veterinary Microbiology* 166, 299–303.

Topical therapy for dermatophytosis

Cafarchia, C., Figueredo, L.A. and Otranto, D. (2013) Fungal diseases of horses. *Veterinary Microbiology* 167, 215–234.

Mayer, H. (1983) [Therapy of dermatomycoses in the horse.] *Berliner und Münchener Tierärztliche Wochenschrift* 96, 458–459.

Rochette, F., Engelen, M. and Vanden Bossche, H. (2003) Antifungal agents of use in animal health – practical applications. *Journal of Veterinary Pharmacology and Therapeutics* 26, 31–53.

Topical therapy for parasites

Littlewood, J.D., Rose, J.F. and Paterson, S. (1995) Oral ivermectin paste for the treatment of chorioptic mange in horses. *Veterinary Record* 137, 661–663.

Paterson, S, and Coumbe, K. (2009) An open study to evaluate topical treatment of equine chorioptic mange with shampooing and lime sulphur solution. *Veterinary Dermatology* 20, 623–629.

Rendle, D.I., Cottle, H.J., Love, S. and Hughes K.J. (2007) Comparative study of doramectin and fipronil in the treatment of equine chorioptic mange. *Veterinary Record* 161, 335–338.

Rufenacht, S., Roosje, P.J., Sager, H., Doherr, M.G., Straub, R. *et al.* (2011) Combined moxidectin and environmental therapy do not eliminate *Chorioptes bovis* infestation in heavily feathered horses. *Veterinary Dermatology* 22, 17–23.

Ural, K., Ulutas, B. and Kar, S. (2008) Eprinomectin treatment of psoroptic mange in hunter/jumper and dressage horses: a prospective, randomized, double-blinded, placebo-controlled clinical trial. *Veterinary Parasitology* 156, 353–357.

Systemic therapies for pruritus

Craig, J.M., Lloyd, D.H. and Jones, R.D. (1997) A double-blind placebo-controlled trial of an evening primrose and fish oil combination vs. hydrogenated coconut oil in the management of recurrent seasonal pruritus in horses. *Veterinary Dermatology* 8, 177–182.

O'Neill, W., McKee, S. and Clarke, A.F. (2002) Flaxseed (*Linum usitatissimum*) supplementation associated with reduced skin test lesional area in horses with *Culicoides* hypersensitivity. *Canadian Journal of Veterinary Research* 66, 272–277.

Welsh, C.E., Duz, M., Parkin, T.D.H. and Marshall, J.F. (2017) Disease and pharmacologic risk factors for first and subsequent episodes of equine laminitis: a cohort study of free-text electronic medical records. *Preventive Veterinary Medicine* 136, 11–8.

Steroid-sparing agents

Leclere, M. (2017) Corticosteroids and immune suppressive therapies in horses. *Veterinary Clinics of North America: Equine Practice* 33, 17–27.

Liska, D.A., Akucewich, L.H., Marsella, R., Maxwell, L.K., Barbara, J.E. and Cole, C.A. (2006) Pharmacokinetics of pentoxifylline and its 5-hydroxyhexyl metabolite after oral and intravenous administration of pentoxifylline to healthy adult horses. *American Journal of Veterinary Research* 67, 1621–1627.

Systemic antibiotics

Bertone, A.L., Tremaine, W.H., Macoris, D.G., Simmons, E.J., Ewert, K.M. *et al.* (2000) Effect of long-term administration of an injectable enrofloxacin solution on physical and musculoskeletal variables in adult horses. *Journal of the American Veterinary Medical Association* 217, 1514–1521.

Cuny, C. and Witte, W. (2017) MRSA in equine hospitals and its significance for infections in humans. *Veterinary Microbiology* 200, 59–64.

Cuny, C., Friedrich, A., Kozytska, S., Layer, F., Nübel, U. *et al.* (2010) Emergence of methicillin-resistant *Staphylococcus aureus* (MRSA) in different animal species. *International Journal of Medical Microbiology* 300, 109–117.

Strukova, E.N., Portnoy, Y.A., Zinner, S.H. and Firsov, A.A. (2016) Predictors of bacterial resistance using *in vitro* dynamic models: area under the concentration–time curve related to either the minimum inhibitory or mutant prevention antibiotic concentration. *Journal of Antimicrobial Chemotherapy* 71, 678–684.

Tirosh-Levy, S., Steinman, A., Carmeli, Y., Klement, E. and Navon-Venezia, S. (2015) Prevalence and risk factors for colonization with methicillin resistant *Staphylococcus aureus* and other staphylococci species in hospitalized and farm horses in Israel. *Preventive Veterinary Medicine* 122, 135–144.

Weese, J.S., Rousseau, J., Traub-Dargatz, J.L., Willey, B.M., McGeer, A.J. and Low, D.E. (2005) Community-associated methicillin-resistant *Staphylococcus aureus* in horses and humans who work with horses. *Journal of the American Veterinary Medical Association* 226, 580–583.

Weese, J.S., Caldwell, F., Willey, B.M., Kreiswirth, B.N., McGeer, A. *et al.* (2006) An outbreak of methicillin-resistant *Staphylococcus aureus* skin infections resulting from horse to human transmission in a veterinary hospital. *Veterinary Microbiology* 114, 160–164.

Systemic antifungals

Hadush, B., Ameni, G. and Medhin, G. (2008) Equine histoplasmosis: treatment trial in cart horses in Central Ethiopia. *Tropical Animal Health and Production* 40, 407–411.

Williams, M.M., Davis, E.G. and KuKanich, B. (2011) Pharmacokinetics of oral terbinafine in horses and greyhound dogs. *Journal of Veterinary Pharmacology and Therapeutics* 34, 232–237.

4 Approach to Pruritus

Pruritus is a common and non-specific sign in equine dermatology. Many horses are pruritic at their initial evaluation, but this does not necessarily mean that they have an allergic disease, as pruritus can be caused by a variety of causes.

Little is known about which is the main mediator of pruritus in horses. As an example, histamine does not appear to be a main mediator of pruritus in horses, as shown by the fact that hives in horses are rarely pruritic. The response to symptomatic therapy may be different, depending on the mediator involved in each disease. As few symptomatic therapies for pruritus are currently available for horses, it is crucial for the clinician to properly diagnose the underlying cause of pruritus in each patient to determine the most effective treatment option to provide relief.

Pruritus is additive, and many horses, regardless of the underlying disease, develop secondary infections, which can significantly contribute to the development or further increase the level of pruritus. Importantly, allergic horses can have multiple allergies and they all contribute to the level of pruritus. Thus, when approaching a pruritic horse, it is important to understand and apply the concept of the pruritic threshold. According to this concept, any individual is able to tolerate a certain amount of pruritic stimulation without becoming symptomatic as long as the threshold is not exceeded. As pruritus is additive, the more pruritic stimuli are added, the more likely it is that the pruritic threshold will be reached and exceeded. Once the threshold is exceeded, the animal becomes symptomatic. The pruritic threshold varies from individual to individual and can vary over time within an individual. The pruritic threshold can be lowered by stress and is modulated by personality and other emotional factors.

The task of the clinician is to identify as many factors as possible that are contributing to pruritus in each individual patient and to correct or eliminate as many of them as possible to bring the patient below the pruritic threshold in order make them asymptomatic. Figure 4.1 illustrates this concept graphically.

As secondary skin infections are common and add to the pruritus, when presented with a pruritic horse, the first thing to check is whether the horse has a secondary infection that is contributing to the itch. Cytology should therefore be done in all cases (Fig. 4.2), as it can quickly provide useful information on the type of infection and the type of inflammatory response, which can provide clues regarding the underlying disease. For example, the presence of large numbers of eosinophils can indicate the presence of allergies, parasites or an infection such as pythiosis. The presence of neutrophils and intracellular cocci is diagnostic for secondary pyoderma, which is extremely common in horses. Many of these horses are mistaken for cases of dermatophytosis (ringworm) as they have multifocal hair loss and crusted lesions. It is important to remember that staphylococcal folliculitis is far more common than dermatophytosis and that the vast majority of horses at their first evaluation do have a secondary bacterial component. Many horses in warm climates also have a yeast component, which significantly worsens the pruritus. This is often the case for horses that wear fly masks (Fig. 4.3) or fly sheets, where moisture is trapped under the skin promoting the proliferation of the fungus *Malassezia*, for example. Keeping the skin dry is crucial to improve skin barrier function and decrease the likelihood of this type of infection. Once *Malassezia* dermatitis develops, it is important to eliminate it and correct the predisposing factor.

Failure to identify and correct a secondary infection frequently leads to treatment failure when trying to control the pruritus. Interestingly, pruritus caused by *Malassezia* spp. can be rather intense and is rarely responsive to glucocorticoids; it can only be resolved with proper antifungal therapy. Whenever a poor response is noted with the use of glucocorticoids, it is important to consider the role of secondary infections such as yeast.

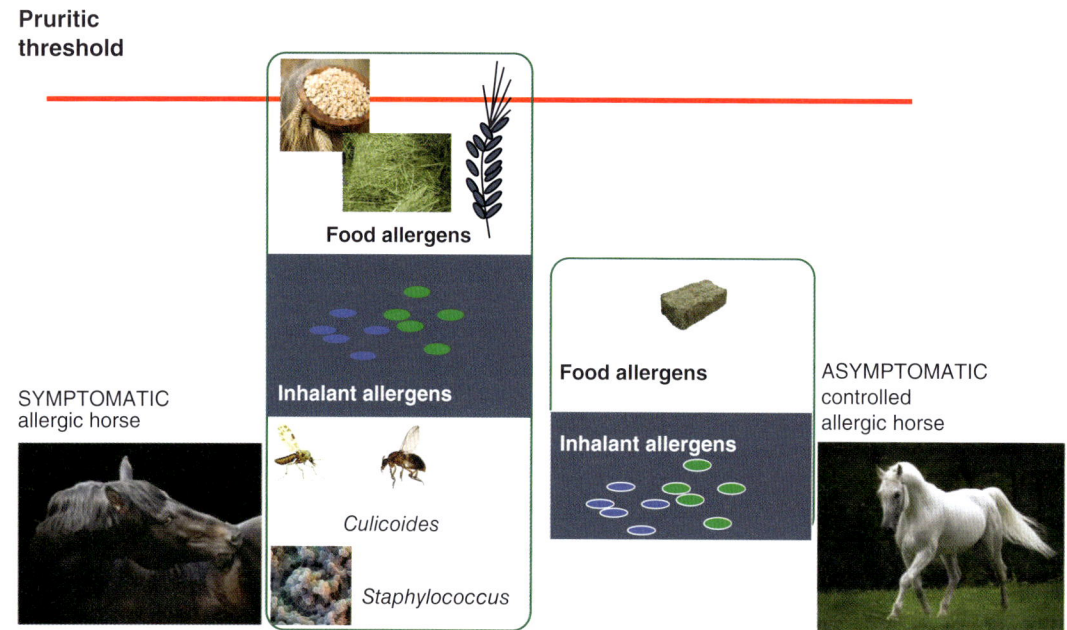

Pruritic threshold

Food allergens

Inhalant allergens

Culicoides

Staphylococcus

SYMPTOMATIC allergic horse

Food allergens

Inhalant allergens

ASYMPTOMATIC controlled allergic horse

Fig. 4.1. The concept of a pruritic threshold. According to this concept, pruritus is additive and is clinically evident once the pruritic threshold (red line) is exceeded. In this diagram, the example of an allergic horse is described. Many allergic patients have multiple allergies (e.g. *Culicoides* spp., pollens, food), and secondary infections may develop and add to the pruritus. By eliminating some of the triggers (in this case, *Culicoides* exposure and secondary infections), it is possible to bring the patient below the pruritic threshold and eliminate the clinical manifestation of pruritus. It is important to note that the allergies did not 'disappear'; they are simply no longer clinically evident.

Initial approach to pruritus in horses

Cytology → Treat secondary infection (bacteria, yeasts)
Evaluate the type of inflammation and note the presence of acantholytic cells

Skin scraping → If mites are present (e.g. *Chorioptes*), treat for this
If extreme pruritus, consider treatments that are antipruritic and antiparasitic (e.g. lime sulfur)

DTM → Rule out dermatophytes in all cases of folliculitis (e.g. crusting and multifocal alopecia)

Fly control → Prescribe effective fly control using repellents (e.g. >1% permethrin or neem oil) to minimize insect bites and interference with the control of signs

Deworming → Consider deworming if *Habronema* or *Onchocerca* infection is a differential diagnosis

Consider diet → Consider a food trial in all cases of chronic urticaria and in cases of non-seasonal pruritus
Minimally avoid high-protein diets containing soy and groundnut

Fig. 4.2. The initial approach to pruritus in horses. It is important to carry out basic diagnostic tests to rule out common causes such as secondary infections, insect exposure, parasites and dietary triggers.

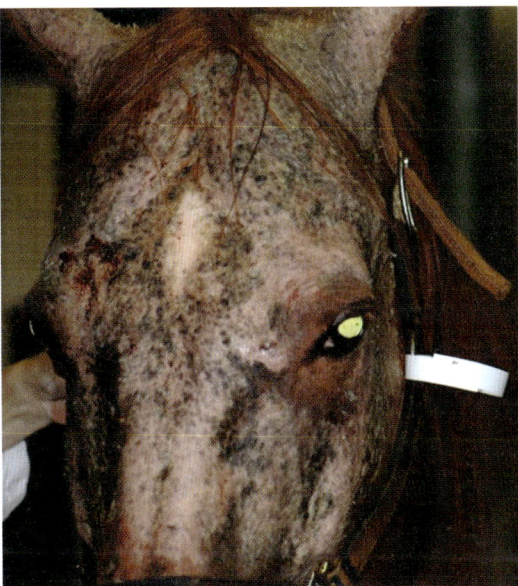

Fig. 4.3. Secondary bacterial and yeast infections on the face of a horse that was left wearing a fly mask for many days while being out in the pasture and in the rain. The trapped moisture provided a suitable environment for these secondary infections.

Differential diagnoses for pruritus based on distribution

Head (face and ears)		
• *Culicoides* hypersensitivity • *Onchocerca* (forehead) • Atopic dermatitis • Food allergy • *Dermatophilus* • Contact dermatitis • Pemphigus foliaceus		

Neck	Leg
• *Culicoides* hypersensitivity • *Onchocerca* • *Dermatophilus* • Photosensitivity • Vaccine reactions	• *Culicoides* hypersensitivity • *Chorioptes* • *Dermatophilus* • Contact allergy • Atopic dermatitis • Vasculitis • Pemphigus foliaceus

Ventral midline		
• *Culicoides* hypersensitivity • Cutaneous onchocerciasis • Horn fly dermatitis • Atopic dermatitis • Contact allergy • Food allergy • Trombiculiasis • Pelodera dermatitis • Staphylococcal pyoderma		

Rump and tail		
• *Culicoides* hypersensitivity • Food allergy • Intestinal parasites		

Fig. 4.4. A list of differential diagnoses of pruritic diseases based on preferred distribution. Note that *Culicoides* infection may be involved in many body areas, depending on the species. It is important to note that, regardless of the primary disease, staphylococcal pyoderma should always be considered as a secondary complication.

When reading the cytology results, the presence of acantholytic cells indicates disruption of the epidermis, possibly due to an autoimmune disease such as pemphigus; however, this is not necessarily the case, as other diseases such as severe dermatophytosis or contact allergy can also lead to the presence of acantholytic cells. This is why cytology should always be interpreted in the context of history and clinical signs. Cytology is fast and inexpensive, and the amount of information that can be provided is extremely helpful.

Mites (e.g. *Chorioptes* spp.) are also a common cause of pruritus, particularly when the pruritus is focused on the legs (Figs 4.4 and 4.5), and thus skin scraping is also recommended in the majority of pruritic horses. This is imperative in feathered horses that have pruritic legs. In the event that mites are not detected but still suspected because several horses on the farm are pruritic and the legs are affected, it is recommended to treat anyway in order to rule out *Chorioptes* from the list of differential diagnoses. Importantly, all horses in contact should be treated. This differential diagnosis is very important in all cases of pastern dermatitis, particularly in feathered horses. As the mite can survive off the host for extended periods of time (up to 2 months), it is also important to carry out environmental decontamination

as well as treatment of the affected horse when ruling out this differential diagnosis of pruritus.

Exposure to insects is another extremely common cause of pruritus. This may be the most important factor in patients with *Culicoides* hypersensitivity or may be one of the many contributing factors. For example, even a horse with food allergy would worsen if constantly bitten by mosquitoes. Failure to take this into account may make the interpretation of a food trial impossible. Therefore, in all warm climates where insects are a problem, horses should be sprayed daily with insect repellents. This is absolutely crucial for *Culicoides*-hypersensitive horses. Many owners do carry out some form of fly control and often are under the impression that insects are not a problem as they are already using some form of spray. In reality, they are often using products that are not truly repellents

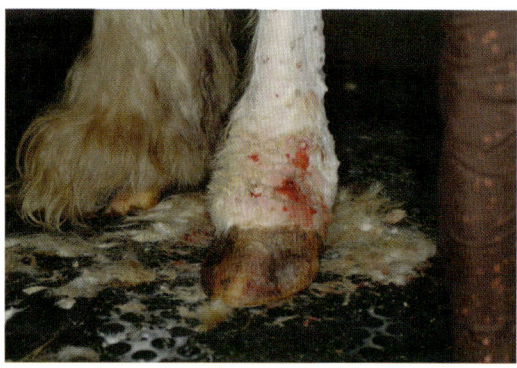

Fig. 4.5. A draft horse with a chronic history of pruritus on its legs. This horse was diagnosed with *Chorioptes* infection and a secondary bacterial infection.

(e.g. containing low percentages of permethrin or even just pyrethrin, which is not a repellent) and they use the spray infrequently. In order for a fly spray to be a repellent, it should contain more than 1% permethrin and should be applied in generous amounts daily, particularly in the summer if the horse is sweating or exposed to rain. If owners want to use a botanical alternative, they can use neem oil (higher than 1%), which is very effective in repelling flying insects.

Parasites should also be ruled out when assessing a pruritic horse. *Culicoides* spp. can transmit *Onchocerca* spp. parasitic worms, and flies can transmit the parasite *Habronema* spp., and both of these conditions are pruritic. Therefore, it is important to routinely deworm horses and minimize the impact of parasites on the dermatological disease.

Once secondary infections, dermatophytes, mites and insects are either ruled out or controlled, if the patient is still pruritic, other diseases can be considered. At this point, it is important to evaluate whether primary lesions are present or not. If primary lesions are present (e.g. papules or pustules), it is important to consider diseases such as contact allergy or pemphigus foliaceus, as these are characterized by a primary eruption. Contact allergy can be ruled out with confinement, while pemphigus is diagnosed by biopsy. Pemphigus is typically not pruritic by itself, although some cases can be highly pruritic.

If the skin is pruritic but no primary lesions are present, then allergies other than *Culicoides* or contact allergy can be considered. Depending on the history and seasonality, atopic dermatitis (environmental allergy) or food allergy can be considered. The classic history in atopic horses is that the pruritus is initially seasonal and becomes increasingly worse, year after

year. Thus, the longer a horse spends in a warm climate and the longer the season, the more severe the clinical signs. Some horses in tropical climates are symptomatic all year round, particularly if secondary infections are not treated when the winter comes. Unfortunately, there is no diagnostic test for atopic dermatitis and the diagnosis is clinical and by exclusion of other pruritic diseases. Once the clinical diagnosis is made, allergy testing can be considered to identify allergens to include when considering immunotherapy.

For this reason, food allergy should be ruled out in all non-seasonally pruritic horses before considering atopic dermatitis. This needs to be done even though food allergy is not nearly as common as environmental allergy. Foods high in protein are more likely to be allergenic. Therefore, it is important to note whether the horse is eating oats, alfalfa, peanuts or soy. Currently, the only way to diagnose a food-related pruritus is to carry out a food trial. This involves transitioning the horse to a diet that does not contain the same type of hay and feed ingredients as its previous diet. Although there are blood tests and skin tests that are marketed as diagnostic tools for food allergy, their positive predictive value (i.e. their ability to actually diagnose a food allergy that can be confirmed with a food challenge) is poor. For this reason, limited emphasis is currently placed on the finding of a 'positive' blood test for food allergy.

Therefore, owners and clinicians are left with the reality of having to carry out food trials themselves to rule out food allergy as a cause of pruritus and dermatitis. Food trials can be challenging when using commercially prepared diets, as many contain alfalfa and soy to increase the protein content. Common culprits for hives are alfalfa and peanut hay, and thus these components should be the first to be eliminated. If possible, it is easier to do a food trial using just hay. Some commercially prepared, chopped hay products are also enriched with vitamins and minerals to be used as a complete diet. The appropriate food trial should be designed based on the previous dietary history and nutritional requirements of the patient (e.g. whether they are actively growing or a competing athlete). The ideal food trial should include a type of hay that the patient has not had before and a feed that contains very few ingredients other than vitamins and minerals. Flavored supplements and treats should not be used during the food trial to avoid confusion.

The food trial should be done once any infections are cleared and any insects are controlled to evaluate whether there is a reduction in pruritus. Trials are typically carried out for 6–8 weeks. If the pruritus does not decrease in this period of time, it is highly likely that the diet is not playing a role. If an improvement is seen, a rechallenge is recommended, and signs of worsening should be seen as quickly as 15 min and as late as 2 days after rechallenge. Rechallenge should be done first with the old diet or previously used hay. Rechallenge should be done with only one major ingredient being introduced each week to enable prompt identification of which one is causing the problem. It is also important to keep track of flavored supplements and treats given to the horse, as they may be the cause of the problem. An example is shown in Fig. 4.6 of a horse that developed hives every time it was given a specific brand of horse cookies.

Ruling out other causes of pruritus is crucial, as atopic dermatitis remains a diagnosis by exclusion based on suggestive history and clinical signs. Although allergy tests are commonly mistaken as diagnostic tests, the reality is that positive results can be seen in horses pruritic for other causes, and thus these tests are not specific and accurate for discriminating between normal, allergic horses and horses that are pruritic for other reasons. This topic will be addressed in more depth in Chapter 5 (this volume).

It is important to note that pruritus can also be triggered by medications such as opioids, and can also be metabolic or paraneoplastic. Depending on the age of the patient and the history, it may be beneficial to consider a biopsy and blood work. Biopsies are helpful to diagnose cutaneous lymphoma or eosinophilic syndrome, which can be intensely pruritic and refractory to glucocorticoid therapy.

Conclusions and Take Home Messages

Pruritus is not a specific sign and many diseases can present with pruritus. Skin infections and insect exposure may complicate pruritus, and therefore fly control and treatment of secondary infections are critical when evaluating cases of pruritus. Once any infections are controlled and parasites are either ruled out or treated, allergic diseases can be considered. Depending on the history and seasonality, various types of allergic disease can be investigated.

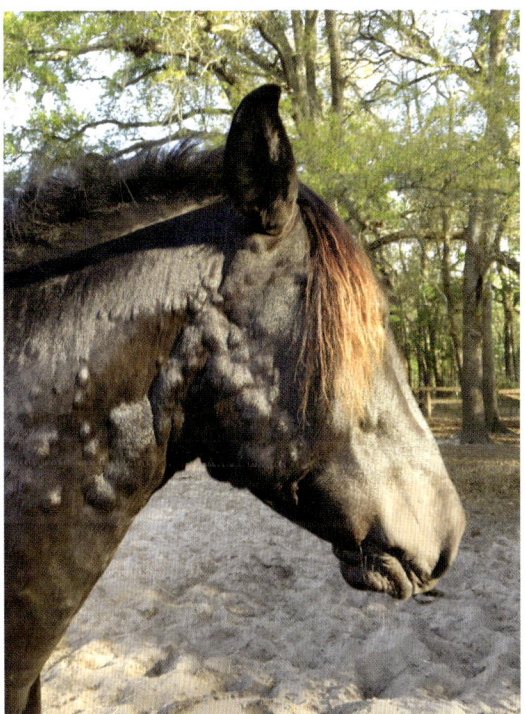

Fig. 4.6. A horse allergic to horse cookies. Severe hives (immediate hypersensitivity) developed within 20 min of ingesting the treats.

Further Reading

Fadok, V.A. (1995) Overview of equine pruritus. *Veterinary Clinics of North America: Equine Practice* 11, 1–10.

Finley, M.R., Rebhun, W.C., Dee, A. and Langsetmo, I. (1998) Paraneoplastic pruritus and alopecia in a horse with diffuse lymphoma. *Journal of the American Veterinary Medical Association* 213, 102–104.

Haitjema, H. and Gibson, K.T. (2001) Severe pruritus associated with epidural morphine and detomidine in a horse. *Australian Veterinary Journal* 79, 248–250.

Jafferany, M. and Davari, M.E. (2019) Itch and psyche: psychiatric aspects of pruritus. *International Journal of Dermatology* 58, 3–23.

Logas, D., Kunkle, G., Calderwood-Mays, M. and Frank, L. (1992) Cholinergic pruritus in a horse. *Journal of the American Veterinary Medical Association* 201, 90–91.

Marsella, R. (2013) Equine allergy therapy: update on the treatment of environmental, insect bite hypersensitivity, and food allergies. *Veterinary Clinics of North America: Equine Practice* 29, 551–557.

Perris, E.E. (1995) Parasitic dermatoses that cause pruritus in horses. *Veterinary Clinics of North America: Equine Practice* 11, 11–28.

Schaffartzik, A., Hamza, E., Janda, J., Crameri, R., Marti, E. and Rhyner, C. (2012) Equine insect bite hypersensitivity: what do we know? *Veterinary Immunology and Immunopathology* 147, 113–126.

Song, J., Xian, D., Yang, L., Xiong, X., Lai, R. and Zhong, J. (2018) Pruritus: progress toward pathogenesis and treatment. *BioMed Research International* 2018, 9625936.

5 Allergic Skin Diseases

Allergies are becoming increasingly common in both animals and people. The reason for this epidemic of allergies is debated, but it is hypothesized to be multifactorial and at least partly linked to a decrease in biodiversity in our environment and to reduced microbial exposure in conjunction with changes in lifestyle and ingestion of processed foods. Regardless of the reasons, cutaneous manifestations of allergies are becoming very common in both horses and people. Depending on the geographical area, skin allergies can constitute a large percentage of dermatological cases and are a frequent source of frustration for both clinicians and owners due to the chronic relapsing nature of most allergies.

Allergic skin diseases have a genetic predisposition in most patients; they represent how the patient reacts to the exposure to allergens and are multifactorial. Therefore, it is unusual for a patient to be allergic to only one allergen. Frequently, allergic patients are allergic to multiple allergens and, because of the concept of pruritic threshold (see Chapter 4, this volume), it is important for clinicians to identify as many allergenic triggers in each patient as possible. It is also important to remember that, no matter which allergy is involved, secondary bacterial and yeast infections are frequent complicating factors and need to be addressed to successfully manage allergic patients. Simply controlling the allergy while failing to address an already present staphylococcal infection may lead to non-appreciable clinical improvement. Similarly, treating only the infection while failing to avoid insects in an insect-allergic horse will lead to treatment failure.

Culicoides Hypersensitivity

Hypersensitivity to *Culicoides* midges is one of the most pruritic diseases in horses. It can start as young as 6 months of age, a younger age than occurs in most pollen-allergic horses. Any breed of horse can develop *Culicoides* hypersensitivity, and breeds of horses that are prone to atopic disease are often also those that develop *Culicoides* hypersensitivity. If horses are born and raised in a warm tropical climate and have an atopic predisposition, they typically develop signs of *Culicoides* hypersensitivity in their first year of life. If they are raised in colder climates, they may not manifest their propensity toward allergies until they are moved to a warmer climate. This is why it is important not only to note the age of development of clinical signs when taking a history but also whether the horse has moved to a different geographical location and at what age he/she moved.

It is common for horses to be asymptomatic for the first year after their move to a warmer climate and then to develop clinical signs the following season. Typically, each season produces worse symptoms that start earlier and last longer, until eventually they may become year round in warm climates. Hence, the classic history of a *Culicoides*-allergic horse is that it is symptomatic in the warm months and severely pruritic on its neck and rump, causing trauma to itself by rubbing against trees and fences.

Statistically speaking, *Culicoides* infection is the most common trigger for allergic skin disease in horses. This is particularly true in warm, humid climates. Many of these horses are also atopic and have some environmental allergy component to some degree; thus, clinical signs of both diseases can be present in the same patient. The distribution of lesions and pruritus can suggest to clinicians which trigger is the most clinically relevant. As a general clinical observation, pruritus triggered by *Culicoides* is more severe than pruritus caused by pollen or other environmental allergens. Therefore, if both pollen and insect allergies are present in the same patient, the single most crucial component of therapy is to control insect exposure. In the absence of an effective fly control program, the efficacy of any treatment for the environmental allergy will be overridden by the pruritus triggered by *Culicoides* exposure.

The classic *Culicoides*-hypersensitive horse has severe pruritus on the head, ears, neck and rump (Figs 5.1–5.3). Horses that have this distribution of

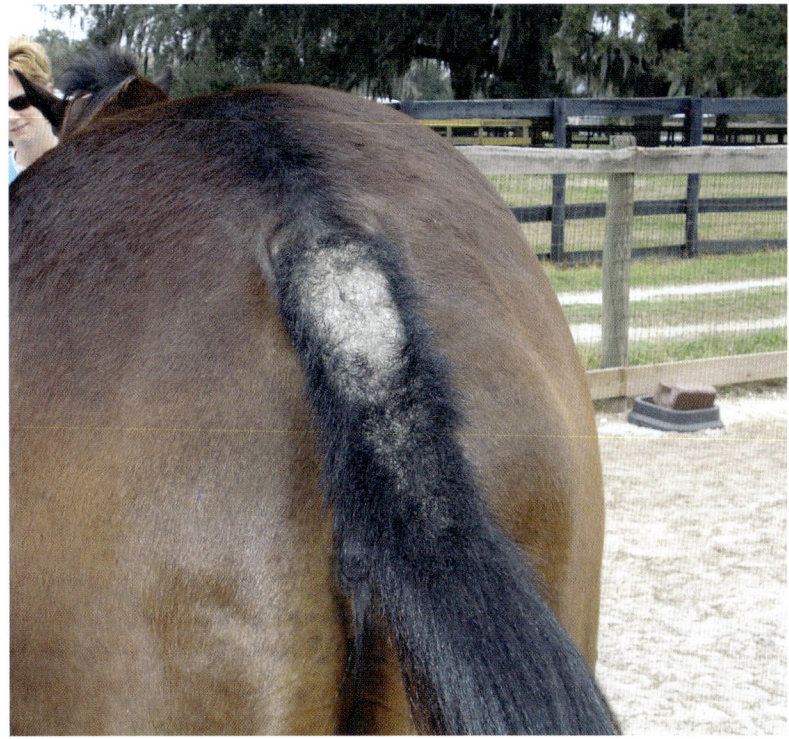

Fig. 5.1. A *Culicoides*-hypersensitive horse with pruritus in the tail area.

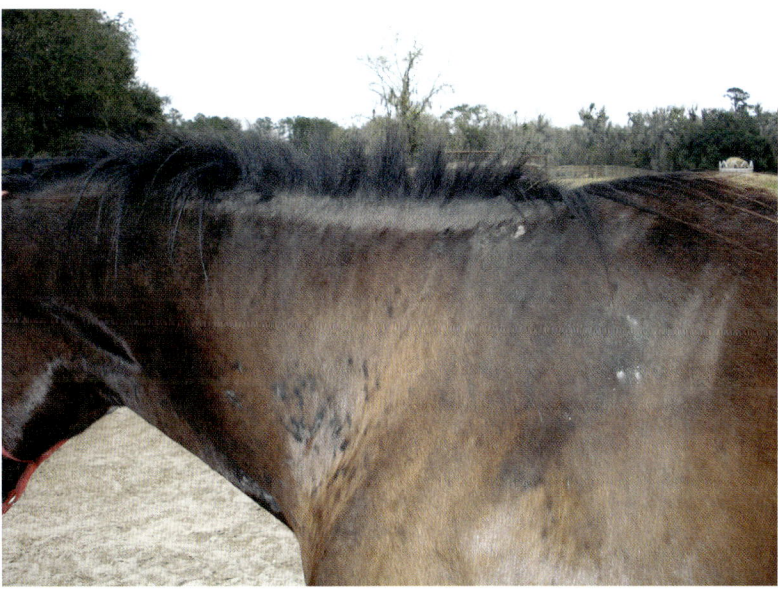

Fig. 5.2. A *Culicoides*-hypersensitive horse with pruritus on the neck/withers area.

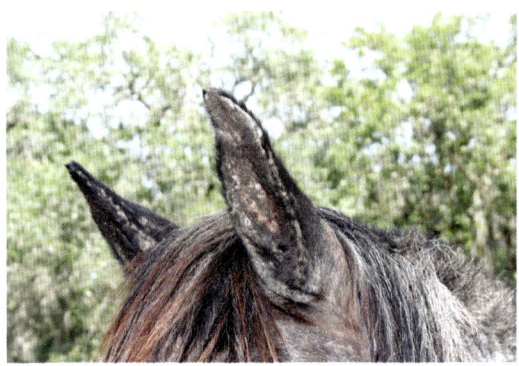

Fig. 5.3. A *Culicoides*-hypersensitive horse with crusting and pruritus on the ears.

lesions and pruritus should be considered for *Culicoides* hypersensitivity before anything else. This is a clinically important point, as many horses may undergo intradermal skin testing for a variety of pollens and may even be placed on allergen-specific immunotherapy, but if the insect component of the allergy is not addressed, any improvement made in terms of controlling the pollen allergy will not be able to counteract the stimulus caused by an uncontrolled insect allergy. This is because itch is additive and the *Culicoides* component may be strong enough to push the patient over the pruritus threshold and make him symptomatic.

Many different species of *Culicoides* exist. For example, in Florida, 23 species have been detected. Different species have preferred feeding sites. Many farms have multiple species of *Culicoides*. Depending on the species present on the farm, the distribution of lesions and pruritus may be somewhat different, and this is why some *Culicoides*-allergic horses are affected on their neck and rump, while others have also leg and inguinal involvement (Figs 5.4 and 5.5). Other sites commonly involved are the face and the ears (Figs 5.6–5.8).

Culicoides require water to thrive and are poor fliers. Thus, the worst environment for allergic horses is a paddock close to standing water. Although *Culicoides* are reported to be most active from sunset to sunrise, in the middle of warm humid summers they can be present all day, worsening at sunset. Horses develop papules and sometimes hives as an allergic reaction to the saliva injected by the midges. Hypersensitivity to *Culicoides* can be both type I and type IV, so some horses have manifestations of immediate hypersensitivity such as urticarial eruptions (Fig. 5.9), while others primarily develop

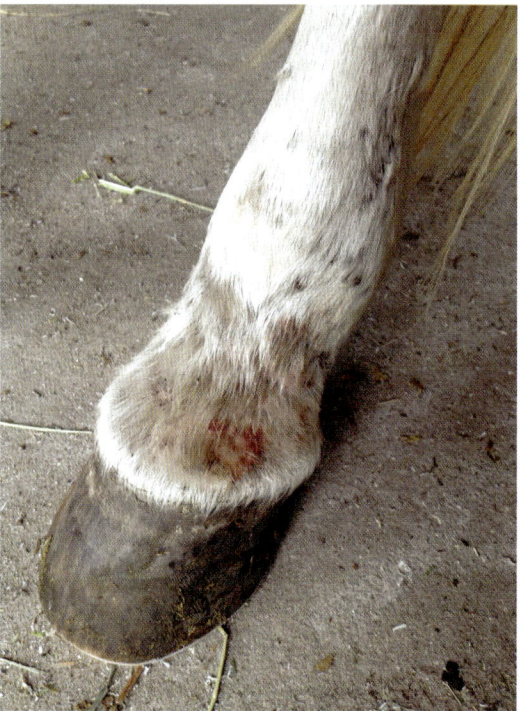

Fig. 5.4. A *Culicoides*-hypersensitive horse with pruritus and crusted papules on the legs.

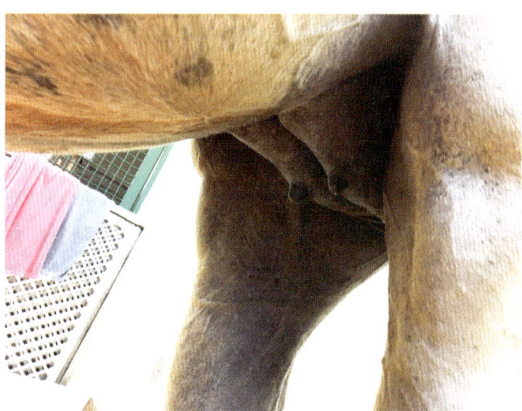

Fig. 5.5. The inguinal area is a commonly affected area in insect-allergic horses and a frequent area for secondary infections.

severe pruritus and papules. With inflammation and self-trauma, these horses develop secondary staphylococcal infections, which significantly worsen the pruritus. Staphylococcal folliculitis manifests as crusted papules and patches or hair loss (Fig. 5.10).

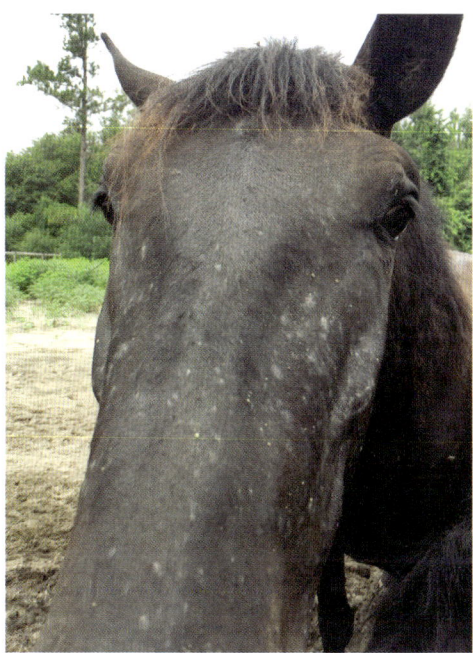

Fig. 5.6. A *Culicoides*-allergic horse with multifocal crusted papules on the face.

Sometimes, the papules are mistaken by owners as hives, but it is clear on physical examination that the papules are solid and do not blanch under pressure, in contrast to hives. Severe hives, however, will ooze fluid, and this can result in a crusted appearance. Typically, crusted hives are larger than papules. Some horses with *Culicoides* hypersensitivity develop hard nodules (eosinophilic granulomas), which have a center of calcification. Most of the time, these nodules are not pruritic, but they can be a problem if they are in areas prone to trauma, or for cosmetic reasons.

Diagnosis of *Culicoides* hypersensitivity is made based on suggestive history and clinical signs. Allergy testing can be carried out, but it is important to understand that positive reactions can also be seen in non-symptomatic horses and that horses with a type IV hypersensitivity may appear negative on serology testing, which only measures circulating allergen-specific IgE. For this reason, allergy testing should not be considered a diagnostic test for allergies in general, and for *Culicoides* in particular. Instead, the clinician should evaluate the distribution of the lesions, the environment of the horse and the type of fly control that is carried out, if any.

Allergen-specific immunotherapy to desensitize *Culicoides*-allergic horses has been attempted in a

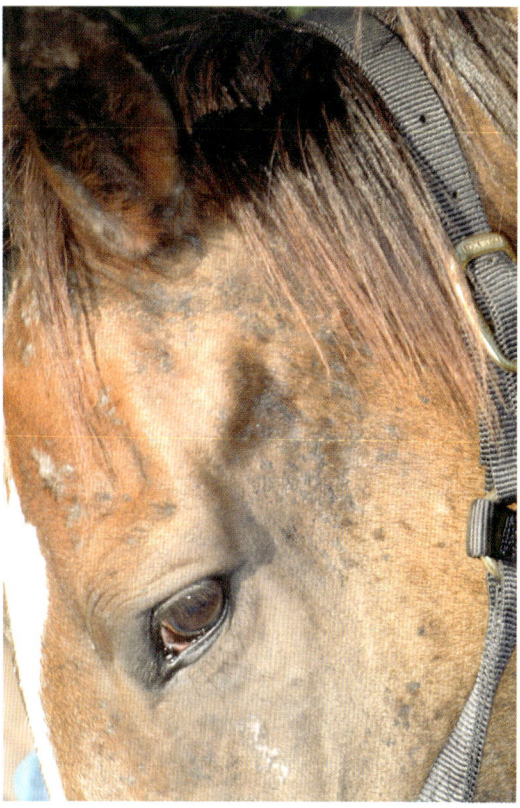

Fig. 5.7. Pruritus on the face of *Culicoides*-allergic horse can be intense and leads to self-trauma and secondary infections.

few studies but was reported not to be significantly effective when compared with the placebo group (Ginel *et al.*, 2014). The reason for the lack of effect may be due to either the strength of the preparations used or the fact that *Culicoides* hypersensitivity has a mixed pathogenesis (type I and type IV hypersensitivity). Allergen-specific immunotherapy is primarily helpful for type I hypersensitivity, and thus insect allergies are not good candidates for allergen-specific immunotherapy across species.

Recent studies have considered *Culicoides*-specific immunotherapy as a possible strategy to prevent *Culicoides* allergy. In one study, this was attempted with both intradermal and intralymphatic injection (Jonsdottir *et al.*, 2015). The authors demonstrated the development of allergen-specific IgG that was able to block allergen-specific IgE and hypothesized that this approach would be protective. However, in no study have horses actually been challenged with exposure to *Culicoides* to verify that this type of

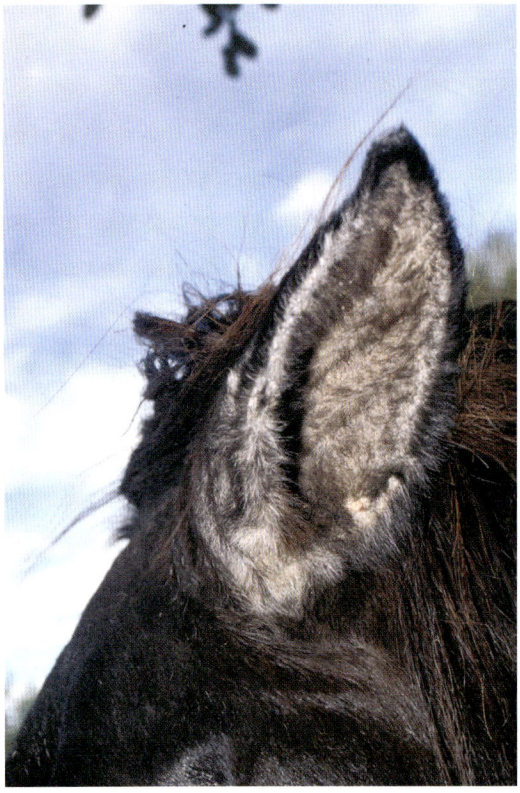

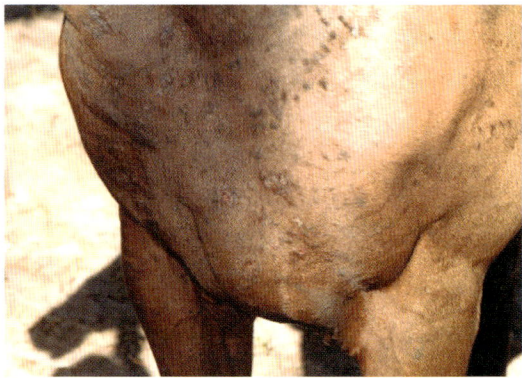

Fig. 5.10. The chest is another common area that develops pruritus in *Culicoides*-allergic horses. It is also an area prone to cutaneous onchocerciasis. Secondary staphylococcal infection leads to the presence of multifocal patchy alopecia with a papular eruption.

Fig. 5.8. With chronic allergies, the ears become crusted and secondarily infected with *Staphylococcus* and *Malassezia*, which further increases the level of pruritus.

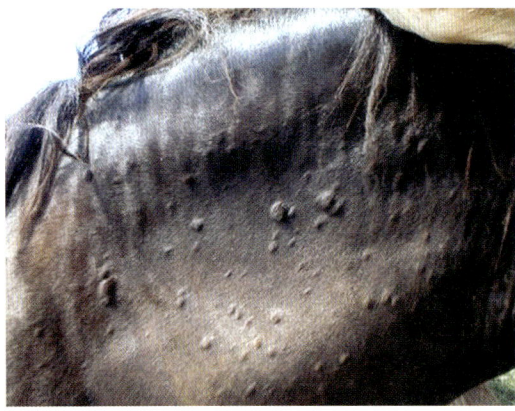

Fig. 5.9. In some horses, insect bites precipitate the development of hives. These horses are pruritic and flare with urticaria when bitten by insects.

immune response is protective in real life following insect challenge. Thus, currently, allergen-specific immunotherapy is not used in the field for either prevention or treatment.

For this reason, avoidance and fly control are crucial in the management of *Culicoides*-hypersensitive horses. Thus, it is very important for clinicians to be familiar with the various products that are available on the market for insect control. Many products claim to be repellent, but inspection of the ingredients listed indicates that they are actually insecticides and not repellents. While this approach is sufficient for the average horse to decrease fly exposure, it is not enough for the allergic patient. Allergic horses need repellents. In order for a product to be a repellent, it needs to contain either a high concentration of permethrin (higher than 1%) or a permethrin derivative such as cypermethrin. Picaridin-based products are available as repellents for both horses and people. Products with citronella or pyrethrin are not strong enough to repel *Culicoides* in warm climates.

The frequency of application is also important. Some of these sprays are labeled as repelling and killing flies for up to 35 days. The reality in warm, humid climates is that the duration of efficacy is much shorter due to rain and the sweat of the horse, and these sprays actually need to be applied in generous amounts almost every day. Spot-on products can be used on the poll, as most owners feel uncomfortable spraying the face and ears. A typical spot-on product contains much higher percentages of permethrin

(45–55%) and can be used once every 2 weeks with special care needed when used behind the ears to avoid dripping on to the front of the face and in the eyes.

Neem oil at concentrations equal to or higher than 1% is another very effective and frequently overlooked repellent that works for 6–8 h. It is more effective than citronella or other botanical oils, and works against mosquitoes, *Culicoides* and ticks. It is almost as effective as DEET (*N,N*-diethyl-*meta*-toluamide) in people to repel mosquitoes, and is a good option for horses that have develop sensitivity to permethrin. Based on published studies, neem oil needs to be used at a concentration of more than 1% in order to completely prevent the feeding of *Culicoides* (Blackwell *et al.*, 2004).

Other strategies can also be used to minimize bites. One is to move the allergic horse to the paddock furthest away from the standing water, as *Culicoides* do not fly long distances and tend to stay close to areas of standing water. Another is to keep the horse inside at night and use strong fans. *Culicoides* are not strong fliers and fans are a good way to keep *Culicoides* away from the horse. Machines like the Mosquito Magnet can also be used, which use various attractants specific for *Culicoides* and significantly decrease the burden of *Culicoides* in areas of up to an acre. Some clinicians recommend fly masks and fly sheets. The success of these physical barriers depends on the commitment of the owner to keeping the skin dry and not leaving masks or sheets on for extended periods of time if the horse is sweating or out in the rain. Failure to keep the skin dry leads to bacterial and yeast infections.

An important part of the treatment of *Culicoides*-hypersensitive horses is to address any secondary infections. As mentioned earlier, staphylococcal infections are common and significantly add to the pruritus. The treatment can be topical (in milder cases) or topical combined with systemic in more severe cases. Topical options for superficial pyoderma are benzoyl peroxide and chlorhexidine. These medicated shampoos can be used once or twice weekly, depending on the severity. An important part of topical therapy with medicated shampoos is contact time. It is recommended that the shampoo is applied to wet skin and allowed a 10 min contact time before rinsing to maximize the activity of the active ingredient. Conditioners to decrease the itch can be used afterwards. These typically are a combination of oatmeal and hydrocortisone. Many of them can be left on. They can be in a cream, mousse or spray formulation. For systemic treatment of *Staphylococcus* infection, it was common to prescribe trimethoprim–sulfamethoxazole and the vast majority of cases responded well. However, in recent years, many cases of trimethoprim–sulfamethoxazole-resistant *Staphylococcus* infection have been diagnosed. For this reason, it is useful to culture a skin sample if the horse has already been treated with this antibiotic to ensure that the bacteria are still sensitive.

Monitoring of antibiotic resistance in equine pyoderma is of great importance as pyoderma in horses is caused by *Staphylococcus aureus*, the same *Staphylococcus* sp. that is present on human skin. Therefore, if the horse carries methicillin-resistant *S. aureus* (MRSA), this can represent a concern for personnel handling the horse, as they may acquire MRSA and carry it on their skin.

The average case of bacterial folliculitis requires 3 weeks of antibiotics. One of the adverse effects of prolonged therapy with potentiated sulfonamides is colitis, and horses being treated will need to be monitored for diarrhea. It can be helpful to prescribe probiotics to minimize the impact on the gut microbiome.

Control of the itch is another important part of the therapy of *Culicoides*-hypersensitive horses to minimize damage to the skin. Control of the itch typically involves a combination of topical and systemic glucocorticoids, depending on the severity of the clinical signs. It is always preferable to use topical therapy wherever possible to minimize the use of systemic glucocorticoids and decrease the risk for laminitis. Topical glucocorticoid therapy can be accomplished by using topical hydrocortisone or adding some dexamethasone to the fly spray mix to make a 0.01% final concentration. Lotions are particularly helpful for therapy of localized lesions such as on the face and ears, which are not amenable to shampoo therapy. For more severe cases, prednisolone can be used systemically at an induction dose of 2 mg/kg/day for 3–10 days. Once the pruritus is controlled, this dose can be tapered to achieve 0.5 mg/kg every 2 days. Some horses may require dexamethasone (0.2 mg/kg/day), although this is not recommended for long-term management.

Other ways to decrease pruritus that do not involve the use of glucocorticoids are antihistamines, although the success of this treatment appears to be limited. Very few published studies exist on the efficacy of antihistamines in horses with allergic disease. One published study reported no benefit with the use of cetirizine in horses with insect hypersensitivity (Olsén *et al.*, 2011). Other antihistamines commonly prescribed include hydroxyzine (1–2 mg/kg every 8–12 h *per os* (PO)) and chlorpheniramine (0.25–0.5 mg/kg every 12 h PO). It is important to note that antihistamines seem to work best when used preventatively before the beginning of the allergy season; they are much less effective once the season has started. If needed, antihistamines can be combined with glucocorticoids. It is the clinical impression of the author that antihistamines appear to work best in combination with other therapy and in patients with an environmental allergy rather than in horses that primarily suffer only from *Culicoides* hypersensitivity.

Another option to decrease the need for glucocorticoids is the use of fatty acid supplementation, although the efficacy of this form of treatment has been limited. A supplement containing sunflower oil, vitamins, amino acids and peptides was tested in a controlled double-blinded clinical trial and no treatment-group differences were found when symptom severity was scored by the horse owners (van den Boom *et al.*, 2010). Flaxseed has been used to decrease inflammation in allergic horses. This supplement is well tolerated and may help as an adjunctive therapy to decrease the severity of the clinical symptoms.

Atopic Dermatitis

The second most common allergy in horses is atopic dermatitis or environmental allergy to pollens, mites and molds. This is one of the manifestations of atopic disease. Characteristic of atopic disease is the production of IgE against environmental allergens that are tolerated by healthy individuals. Some horses have both cutaneous and respiratory symptoms (e.g. chronic obstructive pulmonary disease (COPD)) of atopic disease, while others have only one of the manifestations. The predisposition toward atopic disease is genetically inherited. The disease starts in young adults and it tends to become progressively worse with time.

The pathogenesis of atopic dermatitis is complex and results from a combination of genetic and environmental factors. Allergic stimuli play an important role, but it is now believed that the allergic response develops as a result of increased epicutaneous absorption and processing of environmental allergens due to abnormalities in the skin barrier function in atopic patients. Skin barrier defects are well documented in other species such as humans and dogs. In horses, there are very few studies on this topic, but we now know that atopic horses have an abnormal epidermis, as in humans and dogs with atopic dermatitis. Ultrastructurally, the epidermis shows abnormal organization of the lipid lamellae and the upper layers of the epidermis (stratum corneum) (Marsella *et al.*, 2014). It is hypothesized that this may be responsible for increased permeability and absorption of the allergen through the skin, which ultimately favors the development of allergen-specific IgE.

The distribution of lesions and pruritus in horses is similar to that in other species, with the axillary, antebrachial, inguinal and facial areas predisposed to develop dermatitis (Figs 5.11–5.14). Atopic patients are prone to overgrowth by *Staphylococcus* and the development of staphylococcal folliculitis, which significantly increases the level of pruritus.

Diagnosis of atopic dermatitis is clinical and based on consistent history and clinical signs, as well as the exclusion of other pruritic causes. Allergy testing is not appropriate as a diagnostic test for allergies, because allergy testing can be positive in horses that are itchy for other reasons and in normal horses. In other words, a positive result on an allergy test does not imply that the particular allergen is the cause for the pruritus observed in the patient. Instead, allergy testing should be used after the clinical diagnosis of atopic dermatitis has been made if the clinician wishes to do immunotherapy and wants to identify allergens to which the patient has built an IgE response. Allergy testing can be done by either serology or intradermal skin testing. Serology identifies circulating allergen-specific IgE, while intradermal skin testing detects cutaneous allergen-specific IgE. Currently, there is no evidence that levels of circulating and cutaneous allergen-specific IgE correlate, and thus it is no surprise that different results are sometimes detected with these two tests. It is also important to note that the source of allergens for serology and a skin test are frequently different, which may also contribute to the different results. As a general consideration, serology tends to be less specific than a skin test but is less affected by the use of drugs such as glucocorticoids.

It is important to always interpret the results in the context of the environment of the patient and the seasonality to identify positive results that are more likely to be clinically relevant and more important

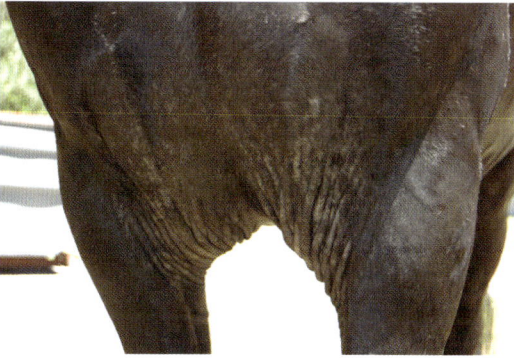

Fig. 5.11. Atopic horses develop pruritus in fold areas such the antebrachial area.

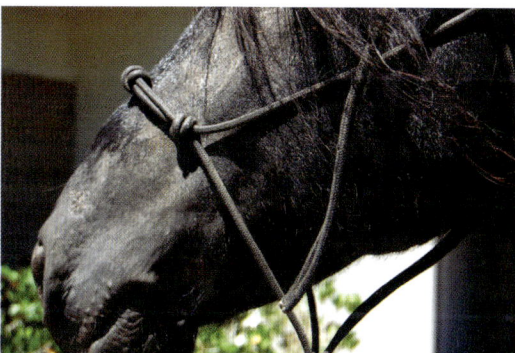

Fig. 5.12. The face and periocular area are areas prone to atopic dermatitis.

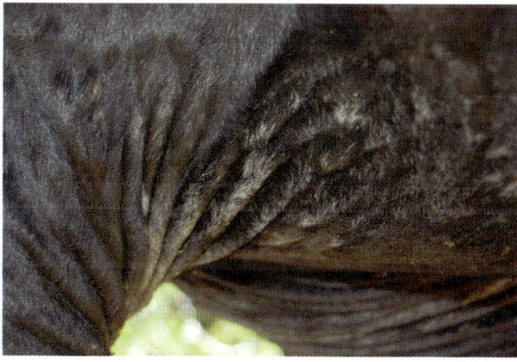

Fig. 5.13. The axillary area in atopic horses is prone to pruritus and secondary infections.

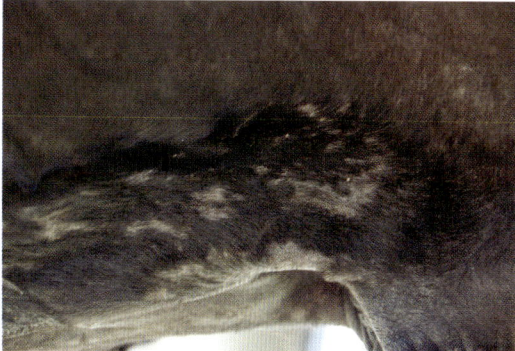

Fig. 5.14. The inguinal areas in atopic horses is prone to pruritus and secondary infections, as is the case with *Culicoides* hypersensitivity.

to include in the immunotherapy. This is important because a more intense or high-scoring result from allergy testing does not always equate with being more clinically relevant. For example, for a patient who is primarily symptomatic in the spring (when the trees are producing pollen), even if they have a strong reaction to weeds, this may not be of clinical relevance if the patient is asymptomatic at the time when weeds are present. Thus, the clinician selecting the allergens for immunotherapy should have some basic knowledge of the time of year when the various allergens tested are more prevalent.

Once the allergens are selected, immunotherapy can be administered either subcutaneously or sublingually. Both treatments have been found to be effective. In horses, historically only subcutaneous immunotherapy was done, but more recently sublingual administration has been implemented, although there are limited publications in the literature (e.g. Scholz *et al.*, 2016). Sublingual administration needs to be done every day, while a subcutaneous injection can be given less frequently; most horses on maintenance are controlled with one injection every 2–3 weeks (see Table 5.1 for a commonly used schedule). It is important to highlight that schedules frequently need to be adjusted to the reaction of the patient. For example, some horses may have an adverse reaction when they are injected with doses from the maintenance vial (the most concentrated). Therefore, it is important to decrease the dose to the last well-tolerated dose. Sometimes, after a few injections of the lower dose, it is possible to increase the dose without problems; however, it is prudent to premedicate with antihistamines 30 min before the allergen injection to minimize adverse effects, particularly in horses prone to hives. Similarly, the frequency of the injections may need to be tweaked. While most horses are maintained with one injection every 3 weeks, sometimes it is more

Table 5.1. A commonly used schedule for hyposensitization of horses using subcutaneous injection of aqueous extracts. PNU, protein nitrogen units.

Day	Dose (ml)		
	Vial #1 (100–200 PNU)	Vial #2 (1000–2000 PNU)	Vial #3 (10,000–20,000 PNU)
0	0.1		
3	0.2		
6	0.4		
9	0.8		
12		0.1	
15		0.2	
18		0.4	
21		0.8	
23			0.1
27			0.2
30			0.4
33			0.8
36			1.0
46			1.0
56			1.0
76			1.0

helpful to give the injection every 2 weeks for horses that tend to flare with their disease if they have to wait 3 weeks until the next injection. Communication with the owners is very important to adjust the schedule to maximize improvement and safety of allergen-specific immunotherapy.

As a general consideration, sublingual administration is considered safer and less likely to produce urticarial or other adverse effects than the subcutaneous route, although such effects can still occur. The main downside of sublingual administration is the required frequency (daily to twice daily) and the fact that more allergen is used so that this treatment will be more expensive than the subcutaneous route in the long run.

The efficacy of allergen-specific immunotherapy is reported to be around 60–80%. Efficacy does not necessarily mean that the animal does not require any other therapy but rather that the frequency and intensity of the flares requiring rescue therapy are markedly decreased. As a general rule, most horses show improvement after the first 6 months of therapy, and some even after the first 3 months. Immunotherapy should be continued for a full year to completely assess the benefit.

As immunotherapy takes months to reach maximal efficacy, it is important to prescribe additional therapy to control pruritus and make the patient comfortable. This is typically accomplished using a combination of glucocorticoids and antihistamines, as described earlier for *Culicoides*-hypersensitive horses. Bathing with soothing and antipruritic ingredients is also beneficial to minimize itch and self-trauma. Many atopic horses are also allergic to *Culicoides* and therefore aggressive fly control is necessary to decrease the amount of pruritic stimulation. If bacterial folliculitis is present, treatment is necessary to bring the patient below the pruritus threshold. If atopic horses are symptomatic all year round, it is important to investigate the role of foods as triggers (described in the next section). Finally, some horses have both cutaneous and respiratory disease, and it has been noted that respiratory disease also improves with allergen-specific immunotherapy. This is the case even in patients that only have allergen-induced COPD without any atopic dermatitis. Therefore, it is helpful to consider allergy testing and allergen-specific immunotherapy in horses with COPD with a pollen component, regardless of the presence of cutaneous disease, to minimize the dependence on glucocorticoids and bronchodilators.

Food Allergy

The prevalence of food-induced skin disease in horses is unknown. Food allergy can manifest in a variety of ways in horses, from pruritus to hives. Some food-allergic horses are atopic and food is one of the triggers of their atopic disease. In horses, some of the foods are also inhalant allergens (e.g. grasses and weeds). As allergy testing (both skin testing and serology testing) should not be used for diagnostic purposes, the only way to identify how much a certain food is a trigger of either pruritus or hives is by doing a food trial followed by a rechallenge to confirm the finding. A food trial is accomplished by selecting a hay that the horse does not usually eat (possibly avoiding alfalfa and peanut hay, which are high in protein and very allergenic). The ideal approach is to use a simplified version (e.g. oats and beet pulp) rather than a commercial one, as the majority of feeds contain alfalfa and soy to increase the protein content. Supplements and treats should also be considered and possibly discontinued as they are flavored and can be a cause of food allergy. A food trial is typically carried out for 6–8 weeks. If resolution of signs occurs, rechallenge is recommended to demonstrate that the resolution is truly the result of the dietary change. A recurrence of symptoms may occurs as quickly as 15 min and as late as 2 days after rechallenge.

Therapy for horses with food hypersensitivity requires avoidance. Currently, allergen-specific immunotherapy is only done for environmental allergens and has not been used for food allergy in horses, although it has been attempted in human medicine. Successful therapy therefore relies on the proper identification of the correct food trigger. This requires a food trial with rechallenge to demonstrate that worsening of clinical signs occurs after exposure to certain foods. Once this is accomplished, there can be strict avoidance of these foods in the main diet as well as in any flavored supplement given to the animal. Knowledge of the contents from the labels of the various commercial diets is essential. Common causes include hays rich in protein such as alfalfa or peanut hay. Soybean hay is also a frequent culprit and exposure needs to be monitored as it is frequently included in commercially prepared feeds making long-term management difficult when using commercially prepared feeds.

Contact Allergy

Contact allergy is a delayed reaction that can develop against a variety of allergens ranging from shavings to sprays or other topical medications. The disease is highly pruritic and is characterized by a papular/crusting eruption. The distribution of the lesions depends on the offending allergen. If sprays are the culprit, the effect may be generalized (Fig. 5.15), while if it is a type of grass, it may only be on the lower part of the legs (Fig. 5.16). An initial way to diagnose contact allergy is to wash the animal and do avoidance. Resolution of signs occurs within 7–10 days. Rechallenge is done to confirm the diagnosis and recurrence of signs is seen after 24–48 h. When there is the possibility of multiple allergens, a patch test can be done (see Chapter 2 for details). This is done on the neck by applying small amounts of suspected allergens (e.g. shavings, plants, sprays, topical medications) to a shaved area of the skin under occlusion. The patches are removed after 24 h and the skin is inspected. A positive reaction is indicated by erythema and a papular/vesicular reaction at the site of application.

Therapy for contact allergy also relies on identification of the offending allergen and by practicing avoidance. Contact allergy is a type IV hypersensitivity and is not amenable to immunotherapy, unlike atopic dermatitis. Identification of the offending allergen can be done by isolation

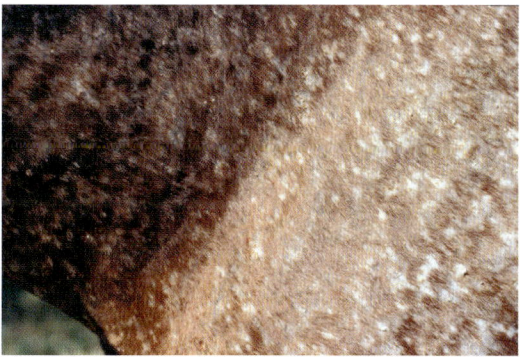

Fig. 5.15. Contact allergy is characterized by a papular eruption with pruritus. Multifocal alopecia is common and is aggravated by the secondary development of bacterial infection. This patient was allergic to fly spray and so the distribution of lesions is generalized.

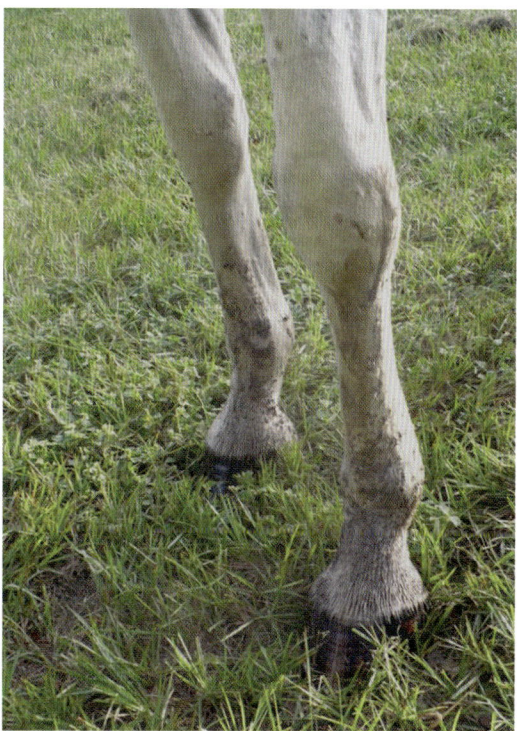

Fig. 5.16. This horse has developed contact allergy to weeds in the pasture. Therefore, the only areas affected are the legs. Papules and crusts together with severe pruritus are the main characteristics of the clinical presentation.

and rechallenge or, more specifically, by patch testing, as described above.

For cases in which avoidance is not possible, it is useful to try pentoxifylline (10 mg/kg every 12 h PO). This drug has been shown to decrease the severity of contact allergy in humans, dogs and rodents. Although studies of efficacy have not been done in horses, it seems to help horses with allergies, including contact allergy. Pentoxifylline is typically well tolerated but can be expensive for long-term use. Generic formulations of pentoxifylline can be used to decrease the cost. However, if a poor response is noted in patients that had previously responded to a named brand (e.g. Trental), it is important to go back to the named brand, as sometimes the response to generics is not as reliable.

In some horses, pentoxifylline may trigger nervousness. Severe cases may still require glucocorticoid therapy to decrease clinical symptoms in acute flares. It is also important to note that shampoo therapy to remove the allergen by washing is an important part of therapy. Mild moisturizing shampoos with oatmeal can be used to decrease pruritus and self-trauma.

Urticaria

Horses can develop urticaria or hives for a variety of reasons ranging from vaccines to drugs (e.g. sulfonamides, flunixin (Banamine), dewormers), insects, pollens, foods (e.g. peanut, alfalfa), water, exercise and stress. Importantly, hives are not pruritic in the majority of horses. This is different from other species where pruritus is a characteristic of urticaria. Sometimes, hives are associated with generalized swelling, which may involve the eyes and the throat (Fig. 5.17). Oozing and crusting can develop as sequelae of severe hives. It is not uncommon for horses to develop edema on the ventral chest and the lower leg while they are in the resolving phase of a severe bout of urticaria (Fig. 5.18).

An important differential diagnosis for urticarial-type lesions is erythema multiforme (Fig. 5.19). This is an immune-mediated disease that can look similar to urticaria. It is important, however, to point out that in cases of erythema multiforme the lesions are not transient, while in patients with urticaria the individual lesions are short-lived. Erythema multiforme lesions are caused by an inflammatory infiltrate, while the lesions of urticaria are caused by vasodilation and blanche upon pressure. Sometimes, it is helpful to circle the lesion with a marker pen

and look at the lesion in a couple of hours. If the lesion is still there, it is probably not urticaria.

For recurrent urticaria, it is very important for owners and veterinarians to identify the trigger

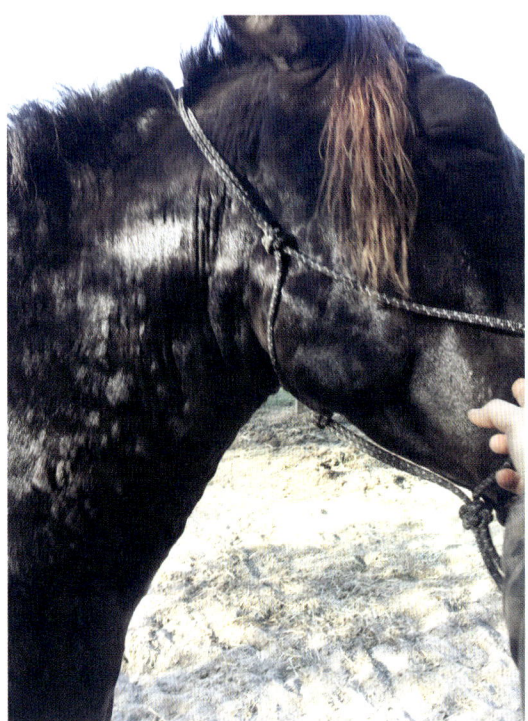

Fig. 5.17. Hives can occur for a variety of reasons and can affect the throat area. This horse was severely allergic to flunixin (Banamine), a non-steroidal anti-inflammatory drug.

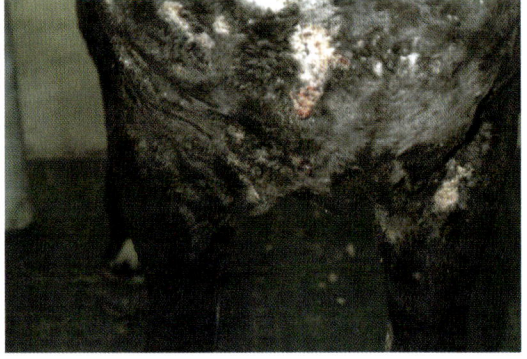

Fig. 5.18. After a severe bout of urticaria, ventral edema is common. In this case, the edema led to oozing of the skin and formation of crusts.

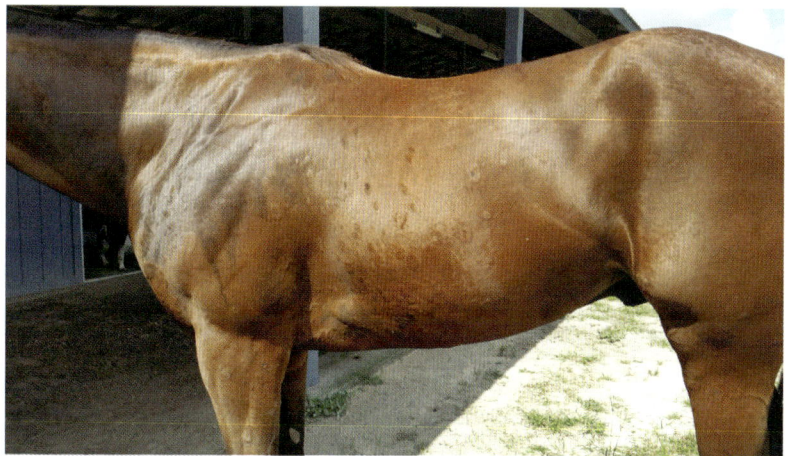

Fig. 5.19. Erythema multiforme can have similar appearance to urticaria. "Donut"-type lesions (with a depressed center) are classic for erythema multiforme. Individual lesions do not disappear upon pressure and are not short-lived as the ones in urticaria.

(typically something that the animal had been exposed to 15–30 min prior to development of the first lesions) to avoid having to depend on medications in the long run. The trigger may not always be obvious. An intradermal skin test can be used to identify pollens to which the horse has developed allergen-specific IgE, although identification of a positive response does not mean that this is the cause of the hives.

Most horses respond favorably to antihistamines such as diphenhydramine and glucocorticoids for acute control of the lesions. The most successful way to manage recurrent urticaria cases is to identify the triggering cause. Intradermal skin testing may prove helpful, and most horses with urticaria tend to respond favorably to allergen-specific immunotherapy. Premedication may be necessary to minimize the adverse effects to immunotherapy. It is important to note that, although sublingual immunotherapy is considered overall to be safer than subcutaneous immunotherapy, angioedema and urticaria have also been reported with this route of administration.

Conclusions and Take Home Messages

Allergies are very common in horses. In warm climates, a combination of insect allergy and pollen allergy is the most common presentation for allergic skin disease. For pollen allergy, allergen-specific immunotherapy can successfully be done to decrease the dependence on rescue medications; however, with insect allergy, strict avoidance is still the main strategy of treatment, as immunotherapy has not been demonstrated to be effective. Regardless of the triggering cause, secondary infections contribute significantly to pruritus and need to be addressed properly in order to provide relief to the affected animal. It is important to remember that some horses may alternate between pruritic skin disease and the development of hives. Hives can occur for a variety of reasons ranging from insects to food to medications. If they are superimposed on another allergy, the hives may be itchy. Otherwise, many cases of hives in horses are non-pruritic. A systematic approach is essential to identify and eliminate the triggers. Failure to do so will lead to a heavy reliance on rescue medications, with increased risk of decreased efficacy over time, treatment failure and adverse effects.

References

Blackwell, A., Evans, K.A., Strang, R.H. and Cole, M. (2004) Toward development of neem-based repellents against the Scottish Highland biting midge *Culicoides impunctatus*. *Medical and Veterinary Entomology* 18, 449–452.

Ginel, P.J., Hernández, E., Lucena, R., Blanco, B., Novales, M. and Mozos, E. (2014) Allergen-specific immunotherapy in horses with insect bite hypersensitivity: a double-blind, randomized, placebo-controlled study. *Veterinary Dermatology* 25, 29-e10.

Jonsdottir, S., Hamza, E., Janda, J., Rhyner, C., Meinke, A. *et al.* (2015) Developing a preventive immunization approach against insect bite hypersensitivity using recombinant allergens: a pilot study. *Veterinary Immunology and Immunopathology* 166, 8–21.

Olsén, L., Bondesson, U., Broström, H., Olsson, U., Mazogi, B. *et al.* (2011) Pharmacokinetics and effects of cetirizine in horses with insect bite hypersensitivity. *Veterinary Journal* 187, 347–351.

Scholz, F.M., Burrows, A.K. and Muse, R. (2016) First report of angio-oedema subsequent to the administration of allergen specific sublingual immunotherapy for the management of equine hypersensitivity dermatitis. *Veterinary Dermatology* 27, 439-e115.

van den Boom, R., Driessen, F., Streumer, S.J. and Sloet van Oldruitenborgh-Oosterbaan, M.M. (2010) The effect of a supplement containing sunflower oil, vitamins, amino acids, and peptides on the severity of symptoms in horses suffering insect bite hypersensitivity. *Tijdschrift voor Diergeneeskunde* 135, 520–525.

Further Reading

Culicoides hypersensitivity

Jonsdottir, S., Svansson, V., Stefansdottir, S.B., Schüpbach, G., Rhyner, C. *et al.* (2016) A preventive immunization approach against insect bite hypersensitivity: intralymphatic injection with recombinant allergens in Alum or Alum and monophosphoryl lipid A. *Veterinary Immunology and Immunopathology* 172, 14–20.

Kehrli, D., Jandova, V., Fey, K., Jahn, P. and Gerber, V. (2015) Multiple hypersensitivities including recurrent airway obstruction, insect bite hypersensitivity, and urticaria in 2 Warmblood horse populations. *Journal of Veterinary Internal Medicine* 29, 320–326.

Mukesh, Y., Savitri, P., Kaushik, R. and Singh, N.P. (2014) Studies on repellent activity of seed oils alone and in combination on mosquito, *Aedes aegypti*. *Journal of Environmental Biology* 35, 917–922.

O'Neill, W., McKee, S. and Clarke, A.F. (2002) Flaxseed (*Linum usitatissimum*) supplementation associated with reduced skin test lesional area in horses with *Culicoides* hypersensitivity. *Canadian Journal of Veterinary Research* 66, 272–277.

Schaffartzik, A., Hamza, E., Janda, J., Crameri, R., Marti, E. and Rhyner, C. (2012) Equine insect bite hypersensitivity: what do we know? *Veterinary Immunology and Immunopathology* 147, 113–126.

Atopic dermatitis

Fadok, V.A. (1996) Hyposensitization of equids with allergic skin/pulmonary diseases. In: *Proceedings of the American Academy of Veterinary Dermatology/American College of Veterinary Dermatology 1996*. American Academy of Veterinary Dermatology, Harrisburg, Pennsylvania, p. 47.

Fadok, V.A. (1997) Update on equine allergies. *Journal of Veterinary Allergy and Clinical Immunology* 5, 68–76.

Lorch, G., Hillier, A., Kwochka, K.W., Saville, W.A. and LeRoy, B.E. (2001) Results of intradermal tests in horses without atopy and horses with atopic dermatitis or recurrent urticaria. *American Journal of Veterinary Research* 62, 1051–1059.

Lorch, G., Hillier, A., Kwochka, K.W., Saville, W.J., Kohn, C.W. and LeRoy, B.E. (2001) Comparison of immediate intradermal test reactivity with serum IgE quantitation by use of a radioallergosorbent test and two ELISA in horses with and without atopy. *Journal of the American Veterinary Medical Association* 218, 1314–1322.

Marsella, R. and Akucewich, L. (2007) Investigation on the clinical efficacy and tolerability of a 0.4% topical stannous fluoride preparation (MedEquine Gel) for the treatment of bacterial skin infections in horses: a prospective, randomized, double-blinded, placebo-controlled clinical trial. *Veterinary Dermatology* 18, 444–450.

Marsella, R. and De Benedetto, A. (2017) Atopic dermatitis in animals and people: an update and comparative review. *Veterinary Sciences* 4, E37.

Marsella, R., Johnson, C. and Ahrens, K. (2014) First case report of ultrastructural cutaneous abnormalities in equine atopic dermatitis. *Research in Veterinary Science* 97, 382–385.

Mueller, R.S., Jensen-Jarolim, E., Roth-Walter, F., Marti, E., Janda, J. *et al.* (2018) Allergen immunotherapy in people, dogs, cats and horses – differences, similarities and research needs. *Allergy* 73, 1989–1999.

Stepnik, C.T., Outerbridge, C.A., White, S.D., and Kass, P.H. (2012) Equine atopic skin disease and response to allergen-specific immunotherapy: a retrospective study at the University of California-Davis (1991–2008). *Veterinary Dermatology* 23, 29–35.

Wilkołek, P., Sitkowski, W., Szczepanik, M., Adamek, Ł., Pluta, M. *et al.* (2017) Comparison of serum concentrations of environmental allergen-specific IgE in atopic and healthy (nonatopic) horses. *Polish Journal of Veterinary Sciences* 2017; 20, 789–794.

Food allergy

Dupont, S., De Spiegeleer, A., Liu, D.J., Lefère, L., van Doorn, D.A. and Hesta, M. (2016) A commercially available immunoglobulin E-based test for food allergy gives inconsistent results in healthy ponies. *Equine Veterinary Journal* 48,109–113.

Pali-Schöll, I., De Lucia, M., Jackson, H., Janda, J., Mueller, R.S. and Jensen-Jarolim, E. (2017) Comparing immediate-type food allergy in humans and companion animals – revealing unmet needs. *Allergy* 72, 1643–1656.

Urticaria

Jose-Cunilleras, E., Kohn, C.W., Hillier, A., Saville, W.J. and Lorch, G. (2001) Intradermal testing in healthy horses and horses with chronic obstructive pulmonary disease, recurrent urticaria, or allergic dermatitis. *Journal of the American Veterinary Medical Association* 219, 1115–1121.

Kehrli, D., Jandova, V., Fey, K., Jahn, P. and Gerber, V. (2015) Multiple hypersensitivities including recurrent airway obstruction, insect bite hypersensitivity, and urticaria in 2 Warmblood horse populations. *Journal of Veterinary Internal Medicine* 29, 320–326.

Rees, C.A. (2001) Response to immunotherapy in six related horses with urticaria secondary to atopy. *Journal of the American Veterinary Medical Association* 218, 753–755.

Rosenkrantz, W.S. and Griffin, C.E. (1986) Treatment of equine urticaria and pruritus with hyposensitization and antihistamines. In: *Proceedings of the American Academy of Veterinary Dermatology/American College of Veterinary Dermatology 1986*. American Academy of Veterinary Dermatology, Harrisburg, Pennsylvania, p. 33.

Volland-Francqueville, M. and Sabbah, A. (2004) Recurrent or chronic urticaria in thoroughbred race-horses: clinical observations. *European Annals of Allergy and Clinical Immunology* 36, 9–12.

Yu, A. (2006) Urticaria. In: *Proceedings of the 52nd Annual Convention of the American Association of Equine Practitioners*. American Association of Equine Practitioners, Lexington, Kentucky, pp. 485–488.

6 Parasitic Skin Diseases

Horses can develop skin diseases as a result of their interaction with a number of ecto- and endoparasites. Often, the skin disease is the result of the allergic response of the horse against the parasite. Parasites play an important role in equine skin diseases, particularly in warm and humid climates. The primary ectoparasites causing skin diseases in horses are insects such as *Culicoides* spp., houseflies, stable flies, mosquitoes and, to a lesser extent, horse and deer flies. Ticks, lice and mites are also ectoparasites that can affect horses. *Culicoides* and flies transmit other parasites such as *Onchocerca* and *Habronema* spp., respectively and these parasites are a common trigger for skin disease in horses. *Habronema*, in particular, can cause severe allergic reactions with major tissue damage, recurrent sores and significant pruritus.

Insects

Culicoides

Culicoides spp. are very small biting midges that are particularly active from dusk to dawn and breed in standing water such as ponds and lakes. They are poor fliers, flying only for short distances and not against the wind. More than 1000 *Culicoides* spp. have been described, and in warm humid regions more than 30–40 species may be active at any one time. The abundance of *Culicoides* is responsible for the variety of clinical syndromes associated with this disease, as different species have different preferred feeding sites. *Culicoides* bites and the resulting hypersensitivity are a common cause of ventral midline dermatitis in horses.

It is common to have more than one *Culicoides* sp. feeding on one horse and, depending on the species involved, the distribution of the lesions may be primarily ventral or may be more generalized to include the lower limbs, dorsal areas, ears, face, neck and rump. *Culicoides* hypersensitivity is considered a mix of both type I and type IV hypersensitivity reactions against several antigens present in the saliva of *Culidoides*. The lesions consist of papules that crust over and can induce severe pruritus, and frequently lead to secondary bacterial infections.

Culicoides hypersensitivity is considered one of the most common causes of severe pruritus in horses (see Chapter 5, this volume). Besides inducing hypersensitivity, *Culicoides* transmit many infectious agents, including but not limited to *Onchocerca*, bluetongue virus and African horse sickness virus. Diagnosis of *Culicoides* hypersensitivity is made on the basis of clinical signs, history (in most regions, this is a seasonal dermatitis seen only in the warmer months), lifestyle (horse in the pasture at peak feeding times in paddocks close to standing water) and inconsistent use of fly repellents. Allergy testing can be considered to confirm a clinical suspicion, but it is important to note that normal horses may also show positive results on both intradermal and serology testing (see Chapter 5). Thus, the detection of allergen-specific IgE indicates exposure and the production of IgE but does not necessarily confirm causation by *Culicoides*, of clinical signs. Conversely, some allergic horses may have a negative immediate reaction to intradermal injection of *Culicoides* allergen. Such horses may have a type IV hypersensitivity, which will only be evident 24–48 h after the test. Therefore, the results of allergy testing must be interpreted in conjunction with the history and clinical signs. The ultimate diagnosis relies on resolution of or a reduction in clinical signs in response to aggressive insect control.

Treatment of dermatitis caused by *Culicoides* involves the use of fly repellents to prevent additional bites and reduction of inflammation by the use of either topical or systemic glucocorticoids, depending on the severity of the inflammation. Although many products on the market are labeled as fly repellents, the majority are insecticides and not true repellents. True repellent activity against biting insects requires high concentrations of permethrin, which is crucial to provide relief to hypersensitive horses. Many spot-on formulations containing 44–64% permethrin, which provides good repellent activity, are available specifically for use in horses. These products can be used on specific problem areas once every 7–10 days, while sprays with lower concentrations (1–2% permethrin) may be used to cover the rest of the body. Sprays should be used daily for maximum protection, particularly in hot and humid climates, as the efficacy is decreased by exposure to rain and heavy sweating. Other synthetic pyrethroids such as cypermethrin-containing products can be effective repellents provided they are applied daily. In order to minimize bites, it is helpful to move horses to paddocks further away from standing water and to keep horses in the barn in front of fans during peak insect feeding times. These measures help to minimize exposure to *Culicoides*, as these midges can only fly short distances and cannot fly against the wind. Fly masks and fly sheets may be used as long as they are changed frequently and kept clean and dry. Incorrect use and infrequent changing of these items may trap moisture in the heat of summer, predisposing the horse to secondary infections.

As many *Culicoides*-hypersensitive horses develop a secondary bacterial infection that significantly adds to pruritus severity, antimicrobial therapy is needed in most cases. In mild cases, this can be accomplished using topical therapy, such as benzoyl peroxide or chlorhexidine shampoo (weekly), or topical application of oxychlorine-based sprays (daily). In more severe cases, oral antimicrobial therapy may be needed. A good choice is an oral potentiated sulfonamide for a minimum of 2 weeks. Because antimicrobial resistance is a growing concern in medicine, topical therapy should be tried first before administering systemic antimicrobials.

Flies

Horn flies such as *Haematobia irritans* can cause a seasonal ventral midline dermatosis. Horn flies are blood-sucking insects that lay their eggs on cow manure. They typically prefer to settle on the backs of cattle during the cooler parts of the day and on the belly during the hotter part of the day. This fly is not able to complete its cycle if the eggs are laid on horse manure, and this form of dermatosis in horses requires proximity to cows and cow manure. The dermatitis is caused by the fly bites and is characterized by pruritic or painful papules that crust over and leave distinct ulcers and crusts. With chronicity, lichenification and depigmentation develop. It is common to have multiple horses affected in the same herd. Some horses exhibit intense pruritus, which leads to self-trauma and secondary skin infections.

Diagnosis is based on the clinical presentation and identification of the flies. The latter rarely leave the host so should easily be detected on the horse. Treatment involves fly control by both removal of the cow manure and use of fly sprays, and control of the inflammation and any secondary infection. To control pruritus and inflammation, topical glucocorticoids can be used; in more severe cases, a short course of a systemic glucocorticoid may be needed. In terms of topical glucocorticoids, triamcinolone is a frequent choice. This type of product is easy to use and can minimize the need for systemic therapy, thus decreasing the risk of adverse effects related to systemic glucocorticoid administration.

Other flies that can cause ventral dermatitis include black flies (*Simulium* spp.), horse flies (tabanids such as *Tabanus* and *Haematopota* spp.), other flies that bite horses such as deer flies (*Chrysops* spp.) and yellow flies (*Diachlorus* spp.), and stable flies (*Stomoxys calcitrans*). Black flies lay their eggs in running water. Adults are most active in the morning and evening and can fly a long distance. Black flies can cause painful bites on areas with little hair. Therefore, the ventral abdomen can be a targeted area where bites result in hives and hemorrhagic lesions.

Horse flies lay their eggs on vegetation close to water and can live for several months. Horse flies are very aggressive biters and can induce painful bites that are preferentially directed toward the ventral abdomen. Once the bite has occurred, pruritus ensues, leading to self-trauma.

Stable flies lay their eggs on wet shavings and manure. The adults cause pruritic papules that develop a central crust. Repeated bites lead to the development of a hypersensitivity reaction. Daily application of fly repellent and removal of potential breeding grounds are essential components of the control of these flying insects, regardless of species.

Mites

Four genera of mites can cause pruritic skin disease in horses: *Chorioptes*, *Sarcoptes*, *Psoroptes* and *Demodex*. The most commonly diagnosed is *Chorioptes* (*C. bovis*), which should be considered in cases of pastern dermatitis, particularly in draft horses with thick feathers. Mites are minute acarids that live on or in the skin of the host animal. As mites feed, multiply and die, they injure the host's skin. Lesions may occur as a result of mechanical damage, secretion of irritant substances by the mite, immunological hypersensitivity to the foreign antigens of the mite or secondary infection. Life cycles are generally 14–28 days (depending on conditions) and the majority of time is spent on the host. Pruritus damages the skin, which promotes the development of bacterial infections. Transmission is mainly by direct contact, although occasionally from the environment or fomites.

The primary clinical lesion is a papule. The location of the lesions is usually characteristic of the particular species of mite, especially in the early stages. The extent of the lesions depends on the number of mites, their reproductive activity and the host's reaction. Pruritus is usually moderate to severe, although subclinical carriers do exist. Self-trauma leads to alopecia, secondary bacterial infections, lichenification and hyperpigmentation. Chronic infection leads to debilitation, weight loss, stunted weight gain and growth, reduced feed conversion and damage to the skin.

Diagnosis is based on the history, clinical signs and skin scrapings (one or two deep scrapings from affected areas and numerous broad superficial scrapings). Scraping large quantities of scale and crust into a Petri dish with mineral oil, and examination under a dissecting microscope may facilitate finding mites. One technique to concentrate mites is to collect several crusts and scales, place them in a 10% solution of KOH for 20–30 min, and then centrifuge and examine the sediment. Alternatively, a fecal flotation test can be used by adding fecal flotation solution to the test tube and placing a coverslip on top to collect the mites when they float to the top.

Differential diagnoses for a pruritic papular dermatitis include:

- Pediculosis (lice);
- Superficial pyoderma;
- Insect hypersensitivities;
- Allergy: atopic dermatitis, contact allergy, food allergy;
- Onchocerciasis;
- Rhabditic dermatitis;
- Pemphigus foliaceus (autoimmune disease).

As part of the treatment, it is important to quarantine affected animals and treat the environment with a cleaning agent such as bleach. This should include all fomites, stalls and pastures. Treat the affected animal and all animals in contact with them with systemic ivermectin (10% solution): 0.3 mg/kg PO weekly for six doses. Topical products that have been shown to be effective include selenium sulfide (Selsun Blue) shampoo followed by 2% lime sulfur solution (LymDyp) dips (6 oz lime dip per gallon of water), sponged on every 5–7 days for 6 weeks. Other topical options include fipronil spray (0.25%), which has been shown to be effective against *C. bovis*. These mites can live off the host for up to 70 days, so environmental decontamination is imperative, including barns, stalls and bedding, and tack and grooming equipment. The most common mite seen in practice is *Chorioptes*.

Chorioptic mange

Chorioptic mange is a common disease in draft horses. The mites are host specific and do not affect people. They have a 2–3-week life cycle and can live off the host for a variable amount of time depending on environmental conditions. Clinical signs include erythema, alopecia, excoriations, crusts and moderate to severe pruritus (Figs 6.1–6.3). Subclinical

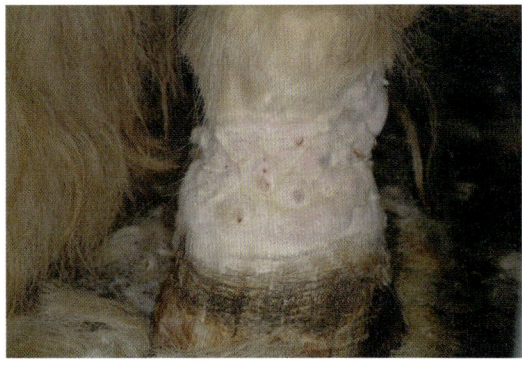

Fig. 6.1. A draft horse with nodules and pruritus on the lower leg. *Chorioptes* mites were found on skin scrapings.

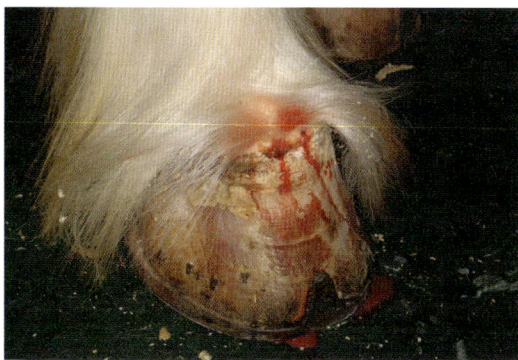

Fig. 6.2. A draft hose with crusting and scaling, and severe pruritus. *Chorioptes* mites were found on skin scrapings.

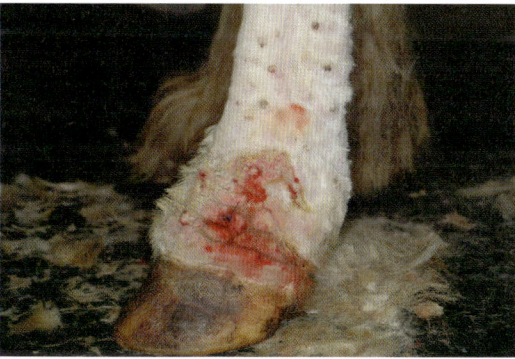

Fig. 6.3, A long-standing case of pruritus on the lower legs. This horse was diagnosed with chronic progressive lymphedema. *Chorioptes* mites were found on skin scrapings.

carriers of the mite occur (possibly as high as 40–60% of an infested herd may be subclinical). The distribution of the mite is the fetlock, pastern, perineum, back of the udder and rear legs. Rarely, severe coronitis can develop. The feathers of draft horses may be a site of asymptomatic carriage. The mite can extend proximally from rear limbs to involve the tail and perineum. Diagnosis is done by skin scraping. The mites are easily found on superficial skin scrapings (note that mites are usually fast moving). Treatment of this superficial mite is challenging, and treatment failures and relapses are common. Importantly, all animals in contact with the diseased animal need to be treated concurrently. The treatment should be minimally extended to

cover the life cycle (3 weeks). In addition, as the mites can survive off the host for more than 2 months, it is wise to extend the treatment to cover this period of time.

Moxidectin has been proposed as a suitable treatment, but in one study, moxidectin in combination with environmental insecticide treatment was found to be ineffective in the treatment of *C. bovis* in feathered horses (Rüfenacht *et al.*, 2011). Failures have also been seen with ivermectin, most likely due to the superficial nature of the mites and their feeding habits (Littlewood *et al.*, 1995). Lime sulfur has been shown to be effective to treat *Chorioptes* when applied as a 5% solution four times at 1-week intervals (Paterson and Coumbe, 2009). Shampoo with an antibacterial product that will help remove the crusts (e.g. benzoyl peroxide) is recommended before the dip. Lime sulfur dip will stain the hair and skin yellow and has an intense unpleasant sulfur smell. The dip should not be rinsed off to ensure residual activity. Fipronil has also been reported to be effective, although this is an off-label use for this insecticide (Rendle *et al.*, 2007). If feathers are present, it is advisable to clip the legs to facilitate topical therapy and better visualize and clean the area. Although clipping of the feathers is very helpful when treating this disease topically, resistance from owners is frequently encountered, as they are typically concerned about the amount of time required for the feathers to grow back. Horses should not be kept in muddy, wet conditions to allow the skin to dry and heal.

Sarcoptic mange

Sarcoptic mange is an extremely rare cause of dermatitis in horses and has been eradicated in the USA for many years. *Sarcoptes scabiei* can affect a variety of hosts, and thus cross-infestation between different animals and humans is possible. Scabies is characterized by non-follicular papules, crusts, excoriations, alopecia and lichenification. The pruritus is caused by the mite itself and is aggravated by the allergic response that develops against the mite. Intense pruritus leads to self-trauma and the possible development of secondary bacterial infections. Lesions begin on the head and neck and progress to cover the entire body. Diagnosis is difficult as the mites are not numerous. Differential diagnoses for this presentation include allergies, particularly atopic dermatitis and *Culicoides* hypersensitivity with secondary bacterial infections. Additionally, dermatophytosis, dermatophilosis and contact allergy should be considered as causes for a pruritic papular dermatitis.

The final diagnosis is made by finding the mites on superficial skin scrapings. As the mites are very difficult to find on skin scrapings, negative superficial scrapes do not rule out sarcoptic mange, and treatment with ivermectin or lime sulfur should be done regardless of the findings of the skin scraping. The ears are often the best site to scrape.

Psoroptic mange

Psoroptic mange can present with generalized dermatitis and otitis and can be caused by two different mites.

Psoroptes equi causes 'body mange'. These mites have a life cycle of approximately 2 weeks and can survive off the host for several days. The mites do not burrow; they live on the skin surface or under crusts and scale. This is a **reportable disease** in horses (ear mites are not reportable). No cases have been reported in the USA since 1970, but sheep scab is still present in many countries, including some in western Europe. Clinical signs include pruritus, papules and alopecia. Scaling and crusting develop over time, giving the clinical presentation of seborrhea. The distribution of lesions includes the head, the base of the mane and the tail base. Clinical signs are more severe in fall and winter. Diagnosis comes from detection of the mites on skin scrapings, but as the mites are difficult to find, treatment should be initiated if mange is suspected, even if the skin scrapings are negative. Treatment involves topical miticidal solutions, in association with whole-body dipping. *Psoroptes* spp. can survive for up to a couple of weeks in the environment, and thus transmission may be by direct contact or through an infested environment. Systemic ivermectin (0.3 mg/kg PO) is very effective. Treatment should be repeated three times at 2-weeks intervals. Topical eprinomectin pour-on solution (at a dose of 0.5 mg/kg four times at 1-week intervals) has also been reported to be an effective treatment for psoroptic mange.

Psoroptes cuniculi causes otitis. Clinical signs are ear rubbing and head shaking; thick greasy crusts build up in the ear canal. Occasionally, the mites can spread to the rest of the body. Treatment includes systemic administration of ivermectin, which is very effective. All in-contact animals should also be treated. Environmental acaricidal treatment is imperative, including the grooming equipment, tack, stalls and pasture.

Demodectic mange

Demodex mites reside in the hair follicles of horses, as they do in other species. Clinical disease, however, is very rare in horses and is only diagnosed in severely immunosuppressed horses. Two species of mites have been described: *Demodex caballi*, which affects the eyelids and the muzzle, and *Demodex equi*, which manifests as folliculitis on the body. Clinical signs are those of folliculitis and include papules, pustules and alopecia. If *Demodex* is detected on skin scrapings, it is important to diagnose and address the underlying immunosuppressive disease. Typically, once the disease is addressed, the demodicosis will resolve spontaneously.

Forage mites

Forage mites such as *Pediculoides ventricosus*, *Pyemotes tritici* and *Acarus farinae* have been reported to cause dermatological disease in horses. These mites are free living and are found on straw and grain. The affected areas are those in direct contact with the mites, such as the face or lower legs. A pruritic papular dermatitis can be seen in the contact areas and, in sensitized individuals, urticarial reactions may develop upon re-exposure. The final diagnosis is made by microscopic demonstration of the mites in the forage or on the skin. Once the contamination is eliminated, the dermatitis will resolve spontaneously. Severely pruritic individuals may require a short course of glucocorticoids.

Poultry mite

Dermanyssus gallinae can cause dermatitis in horses. The mites live in bird nests, and if such nests are above the horse's stall, mites can infest the dorsum causing a pruritic, papular dermatitis. Diagnosis comes from skin scraping and demonstration of the mites. The mites are easily killed by fly sprays. Decontamination of the environment is important to avoid reinfestation.

Lice

Lice are highly host-specific, obligate parasites that spend their complete life cycle (20–40 days) on the host. Infestations, known as pediculosis, are common, but unless they are unusually heavy, they are not harmful to the animal. Young animals in poor condition and on a low level of nutrition are most likely to have heavy infestations. Lice are a greater problem during the winter when crowding may occur, nutrition may be poor and animals have a long coat, which provides a good environment for the lice. Under favorable environmental conditions, lice can live for 2–3 weeks off the host, but less than 7 days is more typical. Biting lice feed on exfoliated epithelium and cutaneous debris. Sucking lice feed on blood and tissue fluid. The eggs (nits) are 1–2 mm long and are attached to hairs using a clear adhesive secretion produced by female lice. The lice are spread by direct contact or contact with bedding or other inanimate objects against which an animal has rubbed to relieve the itching sensation. Some animals remain infected year round and serve as carriers for the disorder. Pruritus and self-trauma result in excoriations and alopecia, and the coat becomes dull and the skin becomes scaly. Animals can become debilitated if they are heavily infested. Sucking lice can cause anemia.

The biting louse affecting horses is *Damalinia equi*, while the sucking louse is *Hematopinus asini*. The latter prefer the mane, tail and fetlocks. Diagnosis is made by a combination of the history, clinical signs and identification of the parasite. The nits are found glued to the hairs, and adults can be seen on the coat. It is important to check skin folds and within the ears. Vigorously brushing of the scale and lice into a pan will facilitate collection and identification. The lice are usually easily visible; a magnifying glass may help in recognizing them. Clipping the animal before treatment will improve efficacy. Approved, water-based insecticide sprays with pyrethrins and permethrin are effective. The coat should be thoroughly moistened, with special attention to the ears. Most insecticides are not ovicidal, and therefore treatment should be repeated in 2 weeks. The housing and bedding should also be sprayed. Ivermectin is useful for the treatment of sucking lice, as populations are decreased by more than 90% after one injection, and has shown promise in controlling lice. Ivermectin has been shown to be almost 100% effective in treating biting lice in calves when used as a pour-on solution.

Ticks

Ticks can cause dermatological disease in a variety of ways. The most common one is by inducing a nodular reaction at the site of the bite. The inflammatory response is determined by the interaction between the tick and the immune response of the host. In first exposures, the main reaction is a toxic one, which manifests as necrotic changes in the epidermis and dermis and a subsequent inflammatory response to the tissue damage. In animals that have been already exposed and have developed sensitization, the inflammatory response to the bite is more severe and persistent. Pyogranulomatous reactions are common and are demonstrated clinically by the development of hard nodules at the site of the bite that can open and drain a purulent exudate. Pruritus is variable. Different types of hypersensitivities may develop against tick bites. Some individuals can build type I hypersensitivity and, when challenged, develop a generalized pruritic, papular reaction. Some individuals develop generalized urticaria and even angioedema. In some cases, the urticaria may persist for weeks after the tick bite. Ticks can also trigger type III hypersensitivity, which leads to vasculitis-type lesions. Vasculitis can present as punctate ulcerated lesions that, in severe cases, can coalesce and lead to the formation of large necrotic areas. Body sites that are prone to vasculitis are the extremities (e.g. tip of the ears and tail) and the lower limbs. Generalized malaise may be present, as well as fever and edema. Secondary infections are common and will need to be treated aggressively. Ticks have the ability to transmit various viral, rickettsial and bacterial diseases and so are additionally able to trigger vasculitis through the development of these infections.

In terms of classification, ticks are divided into soft and hard ticks. An example of a soft tick (argasid) is *Otobius megnini*, also called the 'spinous ear tick'. This tick lays eggs in crevices and can cause severe otitis in horses. Clinical signs include severe inflammation of the ear canal, head shaking and ear rubbing. In severe cases, head tilt and muscle spasm have been described. Diagnosis is made by demonstrating the presence of the tick. Treatment involves physical removal of the ticks and cleaning of the exudate. If a secondary infection is present, it needs to be properly diagnosed and treated.

Hard ticks are ixodids and examples are *Ixodes*, *Dermacentor* and *Amblyomma* spp. *Ixodes* can transmit Lyme disease, which is caused by infection with *Borrelia burgdorferi*. Such infection is common in horses and ponies from the New England and mid-Atlantic regions of the USA. Although horses appear to be less predisposed to the development of this disease than humans, they can still develop clinical signs. Symptoms include shifting lameness, poor performance, personality changes, laminitis, anterior uveitis arthritis, fever, edema and encephalitis. In humans, the early symptoms may also be a characteristic circular skin rash called erythema chronicum migrans. This skin lesion occurs at the site of the tick bite a few days or up to several weeks after the tick bite. The area is erythematous and warm but is generally painless. These circular macules of erythema show some clearing in the center, developing the appearance of a bull's-eye. In horses, cutaneous lesions are possible but are typically missed due to the presence of the coat. Lyme disease is diagnosed based on a combination of clinical signs and blood tests to detect antigen-specific antibodies.

Nematodes

Cutaneous onchocerciasis

Onchocerca cervicalis is a filarid nematode parasite of horses. The prevalence of infection varies considerably in different parts of the country. A high percentage of horses in California and other parts of the USA are infected, although the vast majority do not have clinical problems. The adult nematodes reside in the ligamentum nuchae and form nodules. The females are viviparous and produce large numbers of microfilariae. The microfilariae migrate via the connective tissue (not via the blood) to the upper layers of the dermis. Approximately 95% of the microfilariae are located in the skin of the ventral midline, face and eyelids. Small numbers of microfilariae can usually be found in the skin of most areas of the body. In horses with high concentrations of microfilariae, the ocular structures may also be invaded. The microfilariae are ingested by the vector, a *Culicoides* sp., feeding on the ventral surface of infected horses. Microfilariae tend to be found more superfi-

cially in the dermis during the summer and fall months (*Culicoides* season).

The skin lesions resulting from the presence of *O. cervicalis* microfilariae are controversial and not well understood, although it is believed that hypersensitivity to the microfilariae causes the dermatological and ocular lesions. The ocular changes associated with *Onchocerca* microfilariae in the horse have been studied more extensively than the skin changes. Most of the cutaneous disease blamed on *O. cervicalis* microfilariae in the past has been shown to be the result of either the vector of *O. cervicalis* or another *Culicoides* sp. There is some circumstantial evidence that death of the microfilariae may be involved in the pathogenesis.

Pruritus varies and is usually non-seasonal.

O. cervicalis microfilariae are known to cause alopecia, scaling and pruritus with a distribution that overlaps that of *Culicoides* hypersensitivity (e.g. withers, face and neck). Ventral midline dermatitis is also very common with cutaneous onchocerciasis. In some horses, a predilection for the unpigmented areas of the face resembling photosensitization is noticed. A bull's-eye lesion in the center of the forehead is almost pathognomonic (Fig. 6.4). There may also be pigmentation at the lateral limbus and sclerosing keratitis.

Focal crusting, hair loss and depigmentation of the skin may occur at the base of the mane, as well as diffuse lesions on the anteromedial aspect of the thoracic limbs and brisket (Figs 6.5 and 6.6). The focal, seasonal, inflammatory lesions on the ventral midline of horses referred to as ventral midline dermatitis is related to bites of the vector of *O. cervicalis* and/or bites of the horn fly (Figs 6.7 and 6.8). *O. cervicalis* microfilariae can be found in the skin in this region. Every attempt should be made to rule out other causes for the skin condition such as insect hypersensitivity and dermatophytosis. As a high percentage of horses are infected with this nematode, the simple demonstration of microfilariae in diseased skin is not enough to infer a cause-and-effect relationship.

To demonstrate the presence of the microfilariae, a small piece of skin is minced with a razor blade, placed on a glass slide, covered with a few drops of physiological saline solution and allowed to incubate at room temperature for 5–10 min or longer if necessary. The slide is then examined microscopically

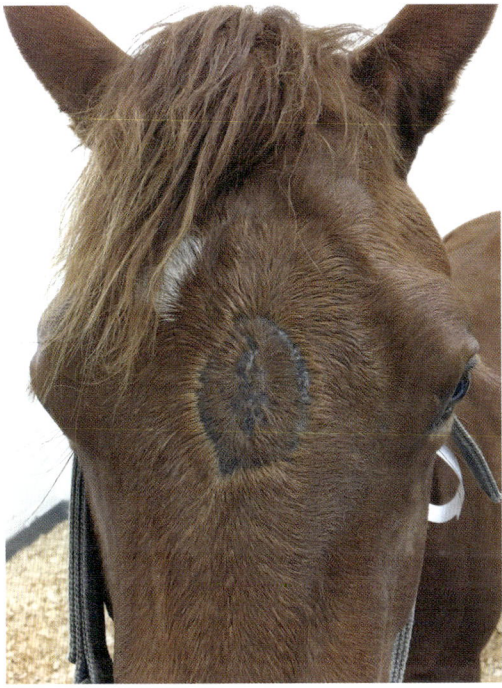

Fig. 6.4. Cutaneous onchocerciasis in a horse. Note the circular area of alopecia on the forehead. This type of lesion is often referred as a bull's-eye lesion and is considered pathognomonic of *Onchocerca* infection.

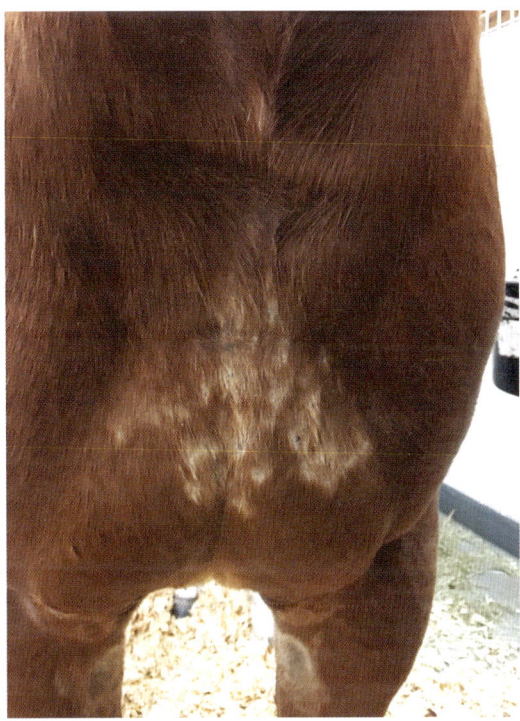

Fig. 6.6. Another horse diagnosed with *Onchocerca* infection. Note the discrete circular crusting lesions on the chest.

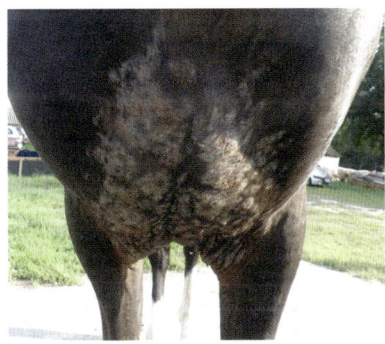

Fig. 6.5. Crusting lesions on the chest of a horse infected with *Onchocerca*.

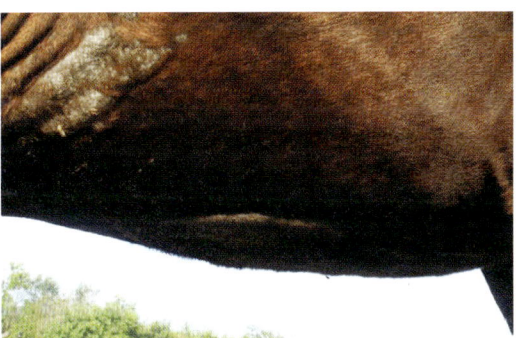

Fig. 6.7. Crusting on the ventral abdomen. Ventral midline dermatitis is a classic manifestation of *Onchocerca* infection.

with the low-power objective. Live microfilariae can be seen easily because of their vigorous movement in the saline solution following migration from the skin.

Histopathology should reveal purple-stained microfilariae surrounded by an inflammatory reaction and a perivascular eosinophilic infiltrate with a nest of eosinophils under the epidermis and near hair follicles. A response to ivermectin therapy is the most practical way to diagnose infection. Eight weeks should be allowed for the response, and horn flies should be controlled during this time.

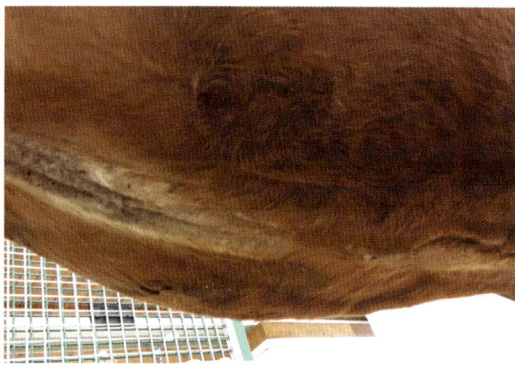

Fig. 6.8. Another case of ventral midline dermatitis. Note the discrete elongated crusting pattern. These lesions are seen in *Culicoides*-allergic horses and can be very pruritic.

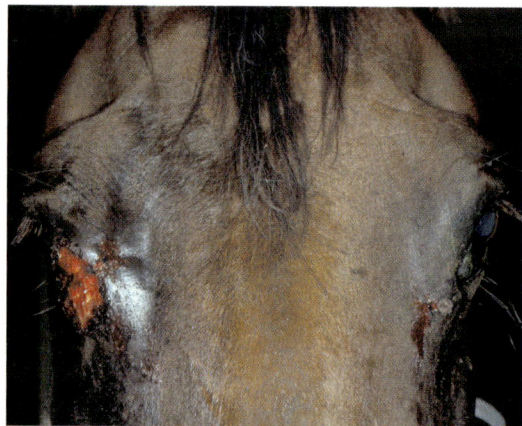

Fig. 6.9. Severe case of habronemiasis affecting the medial canthus of both eyes. Tearing of the eyes in the summer time attracts flies, which deposit the larvae in this area. The immunological response against the larvae leads to a severe inflammatory response.

Ivermectin is the current treatment of choice. It is given orally (as a paste) at a dose of 0.2 mg/kg. One dose is sufficient. The response to this treatment will differentiate *Onchocerca* infection from insect hypersensitivity. Some horses will develop facial and/or abdominal edema following treatment. This is presumed to be an allergic reaction elicited by the death of the microfilariae. Ivermectin is an excellent microfilaricide but has minimal effect on the adult nematodes. Thus, retreatment is required in 3–12 months, after the skin has become repopulated with microfilariae. Systemic corticosteroid therapy is given for the first 3–4 days of therapy; 400–500 mg prednisolone per horse is the usual dose. A clinical response may be noted as early as day 3 or 4 of therapy, and most horses show a good response in 2–3 weeks. Recurrences may occur as early as 2 months after therapy in some horses. Most horses, however, remain symptom free for 6 months. A few horses are still clinically normal 2 years after a single therapeutic regimen (in these horses, the drug has probably had a significant effect on the adult nematodes – death or sterilization). An ophthalmic examination should be made prior to therapy, as death of the microfilariae will exacerbate uveitis, if present. If uveitis is present, the eyes should be pretreated with steroids.

Cutaneous habronemiasis (summer sores)

Three species of nematode parasitize the horse: *Habronema muscae*, *Habronema majus* and *Draschia megastoma*. The adults reside in the stomach where they cause little reaction, with the exception of *D. megastoma*, which produces varying-sized nodules that usually occur near the margo plicatus. Cutaneous habronemiasis results from an aberrant parasitism when the larvae penetrate damaged skin and incite a hypersensitivity reaction. A few horses with wounds develop the disease; once they get it, recurrence is common year after year.

The disease is seasonal, first appearing in the spring, and most cases spontaneously clear in the winter months. The occurrence of the disease is sporadic, with only a few horses in any given area being affected. Once the disease occurs in a horse, it will usually recur each succeeding summer unless stringent preventative measures are taken. The lesions usually involve the medial canthus of the eye (Fig. 6.9), the male genitalia, especially the urethral process (Fig. 6.10 and 6.11), and the lower extremities (wounds) (Figs 6.12–6.14) or around the muzzle (Fig. 6.15). The lesions themselves consist of areas of granulation tissue containing small, gritty, yellow nodules. Donkeys and mules develop very large lesions.

Differential diagnoses for nodular, pruritic, hemorrhagic lesions include exuberant granulation tissue (proud flesh), fibroblastic sarcoid, squamous cell carcinoma, pythiosis (phycomycosis)

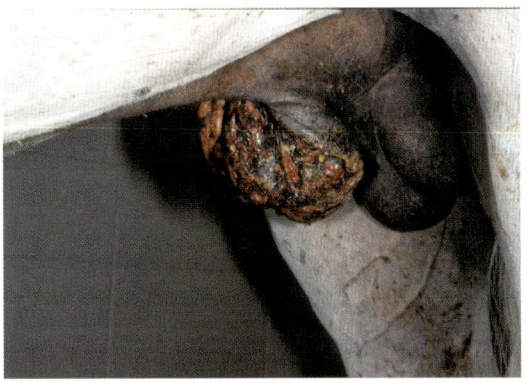

Fig. 6.10. Severe habronemiasis on the penis of a gelding.

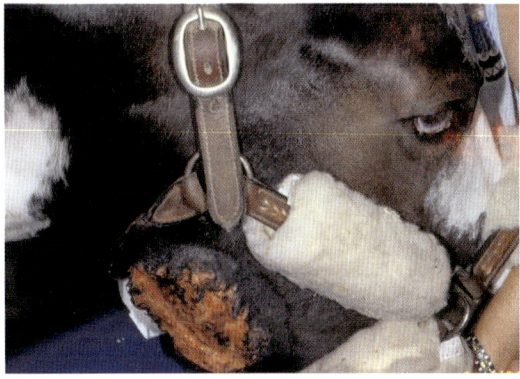

Fig. 6.13. Severe *Habronema* infection on the cheek of a horse. This horse had a small cut in this area prior to the development of habronemiasis.

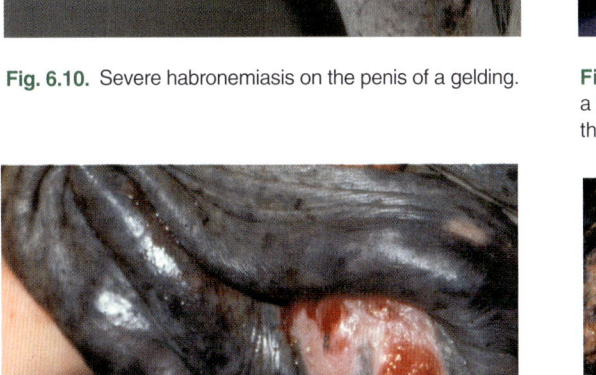

Fig. 6.11. A milder case of habronemiasis on the mucous membrane of the genitalia.

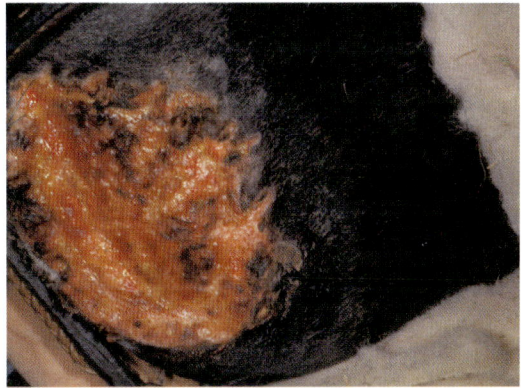

Fig. 6.14. Close-up of the horse in Fig. 6.13. Severe pruritus was present in this case.

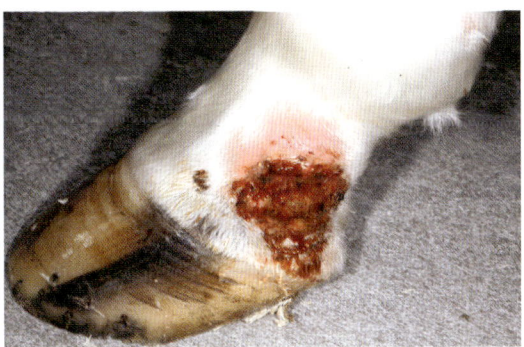

Fig. 6.12. *Habronema* infection of the pastern. Infection typically occurs in areas where some trauma has occurred and flies have deposited their larvae on the open wound.

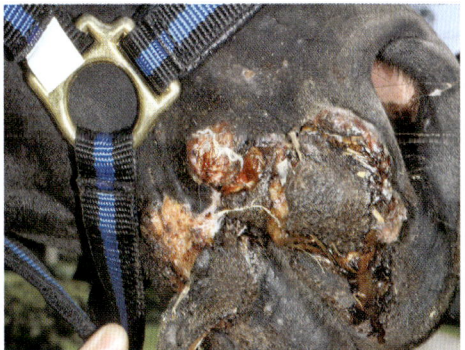

Fig. 6.15. *Habronema* infection on the face of a horse. Prior attempts had been made to surgically resect the lesions. Scarring and recurrence of the lesions contributed to the presentation shown.

and zygomycosis. Diagnosis of *Habronema* infection is frequently clinical based on the history and clinical presentation, and is then confirmed by histopathology. Sometimes, parasites encased in degenerated collagen are macroscopically visible in the tissue (Figs 6.16 and 6.17). Cytology reveals large numbers of eosinophils due to the allergic response against the parasite.

Histopathology of the lesions reveals a severe eosinophilic infiltrate that surrounds the larvae (Figs 6.18–6.20).

The goals of treatment are to reduce the size of the lesion, reduce the inflammation and prevent reinfection. Killing the larvae may not be important as they will die anyway (larval death may be part of pathogenesis) and the host reaction

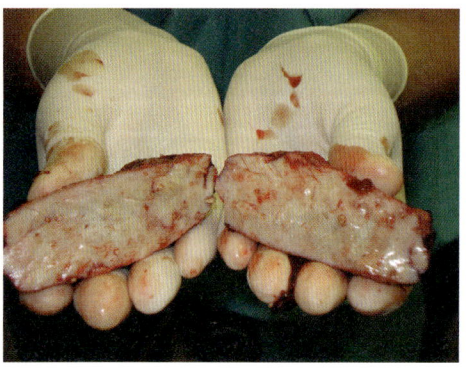

Fig. 6.16. Tissue surgically resected from a horse with habronemiasis. Note the larvae embedded in the severe inflammatory response.

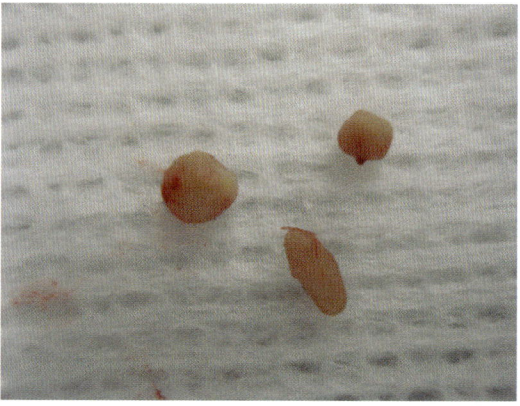

Fig. 6.17. Larvae extracted from the tissue surgically resected from the horse in Fig. 6.16.

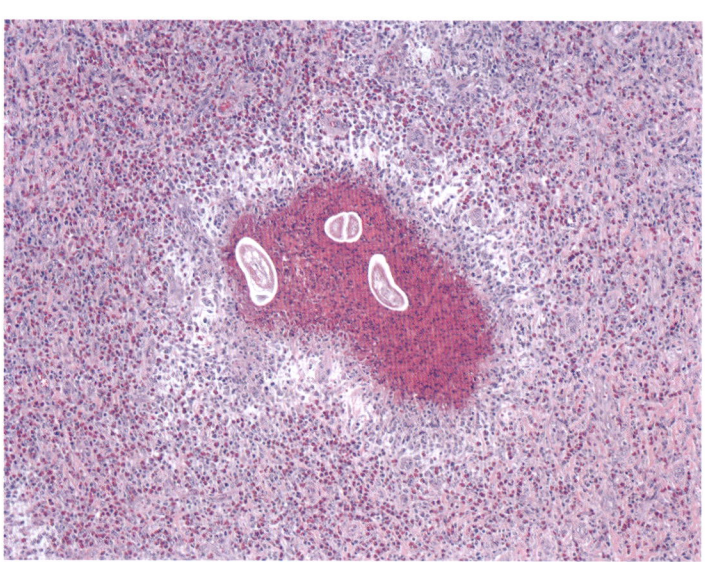

Fig. 6.18. Histopathology of tissue removed from a horse diagnosed with habronemiasis. Note the severe eosinophilic response surrounding the larvae of the parasite (100× magnification). The severe eosinophilic inflammation is responsible for the intense pruritus and tissue damage in the area where the larvae are present. Inflammation persists even after the larvae are dead, requiring physical removal of the larvae.

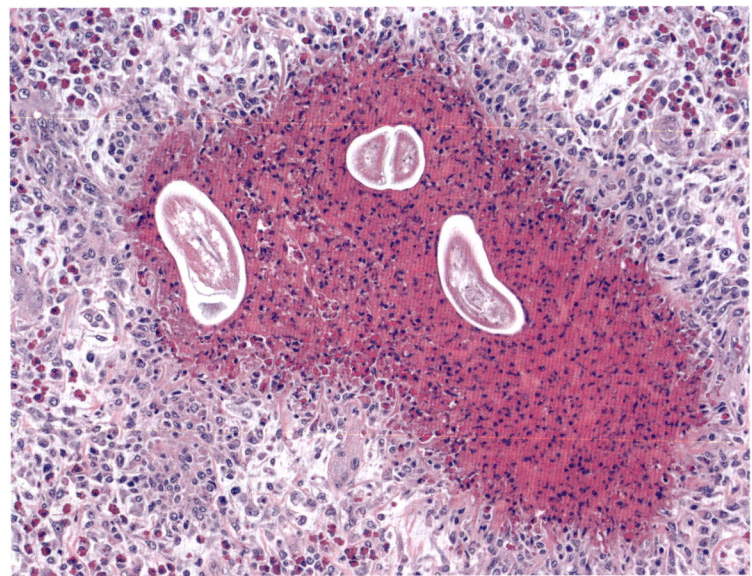

Fig. 6.19. Close-up (200× magnification) of the lesion shown in Fig. 6.18.

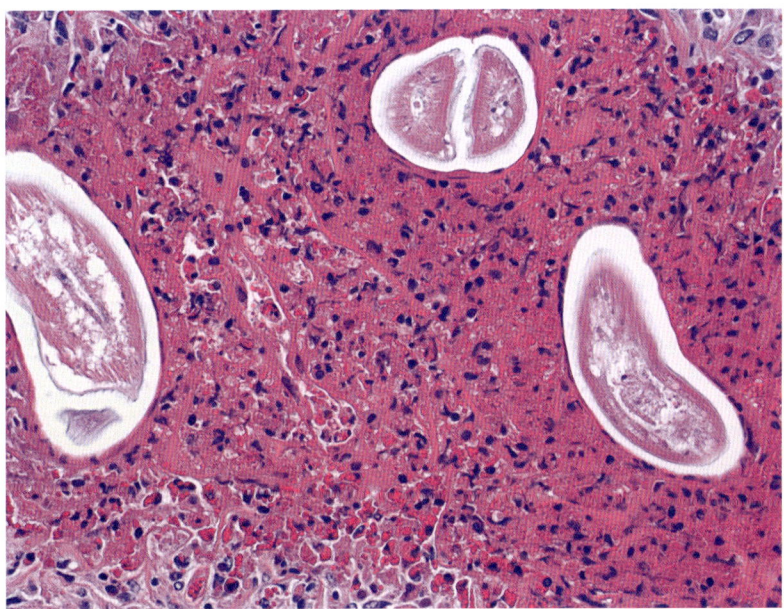

Fig. 6.20. Close-up (400× magnification) of the lesion shown in Fig. 6.18.

continues even when the parasite is dead. Due to the recurrent nature of the disease, strict attention to fly control and immediate wound care should be exercised in future years to decrease the chances of reinfection. Treatment should consist of systemic ivermectin combined with surgical debulking and intralesional or systemically administered corticosteroids to reduce the inflammation.

References

Littlewood, J.D., Rose, J.F. and Paterson, S. (1995) Oral ivermectin paste for the treatment of chorioptic mange in horses. *Veterinary Record* 137, 661–663.

Paterson, S. and Coumbe, K. (2009) An open study to evaluate topical treatment of equine chorioptic mange with shampooing and lime sulphur solution. *Veterinary Dermatology* 20, 623–629.

Rendle, D.I., Cottle, H.J., Love, S. and Hughes, K.J. (2007) Comparative study of doramectin and fipronil in the treatment of equine chorioptic mange. *Veterinary Record* 161, 335–338.

Rüfenacht, S., Roosje, P.J., Sager, H., Doherr, M.G., Straub, R. *et al.* (2011) Combined moxidectin and environmental therapy do not eliminate *Chorioptes bovis* infestation in heavily feathered horses. *Veterinary Dermatology* 22, 17–23.

Further Reading

Braverman, Y. and Chizov-Ginzburg, A. (1998) Duration of repellency of various synthetic and plant-derived preparations for *Culicoides imicola*, the vector of African horse sickness virus. *Archives of Virology* 14, 165–174.

de Raat, I.J., van den Boom, R., van Poppel, M. and van Oldruitenborgh-Oosterbaan, M.M. (2008) The effect of a topical insecticide containing permethrin on the number of *Culicoides* midges caught near horses with and without insect bite hypersensitivity in the Netherlands. *Tijdschrift Voor Diergeneeskunde* 133, 838–842.

Papadopoulos, E., Rowlinson, M., Bartram, D., Carpenter, S., Mellor, P. and Wall, R. (2010) Treatment of horses with cypermethrin against the biting flies *Culicoides nubeculosus*, *Aedes aegypti* and *Culex quinquefasciatus*. *Veterinary Parasitology* 169, 165–171.

Ural, K., Ulutas, B. and Kar, S. (2008) Eprinomectin treatment of psoroptic mange in hunter/jumper and dressage horses: a prospective, randomized, double-blinded, placebo-controlled clinical trial. *Veterinary Parasitology* 156, 353–357.

7 Clinical Approach to Crusting Diseases

Crusting is a common clinical presentation of skin disease in horses. Crusts and scales are secondary lesions, and therefore it is important to identify the early, primary lesions that are responsible for the formation of the crusts, if possible. Crusting dermatitis may be the consequence of a pustular disease (the most common situation) or may be due to a primary disease of keratinization. When pustular diseases are the cause of the crusting and scales, the crusts are typically smaller compared with the thicker and more tightly adherent crusts caused by a primary disease of keratinization (e.g. a disease in which the differentiation of keratinization is altered and desquamation does not occur normally, leading to accumulation of more tightly adherent thicker crusts). Primary diseases of keratinization can be localized to one region and are evident early on in life; they are often asymptomatic and more cosmetic in nature.

The term seborrhea is frequently used to describe a patient that presents with a crusting dermatitis. This term is simply a description and should not be misinterpreted as synonymous for a disease of keratinization (e.g. primary seborrhea). It important to point out that the vast majority of seborrhea cases are secondary, and seborrhea can occur for a variety of reasons from infectious causes to autoimmune, from nutritional to environmental, and from neoplastic to metabolic. Therefore, it is very important for clinicians to address, if at all possible, the primary cause that is leading to the seborrhea. Seborrhea can be further described based on the clinical appearance into dry or greasy. This does not necessarily have a strong implication toward the underlying cause.

Clinically speaking, pustular diseases are by far the most common cause of crusting dermatitis. Pustules can be follicular or not (Table 7.1). Causes of follicular pustules in horses are bacterial infections such as staphylococcal pyoderma, fungal infections such as dermatophytosis (*Trichophyton* spp. being the most common dermatophyte) or mites such as

Demodex spp. In terms of non-follicular pustular diseases, the cause may be bacterial (e.g. *Dermatophilus* spp.), parasitic (e.g. *Chorioptes* spp.), autoimmune such as pemphigus foliaceus, allergic such as insects and contact allergy, or viral. Thus, the initial work-up of a horse presenting with crusting and/or pustules should include cytology, skin scraping and a fungal culture using DTM. Skin cytology provides useful information regarding the type of exudate and the presence of organisms and acantholytic cells. If bacteria and yeasts are found, they need to be treated accordingly. Once infections (and/or mites, depending on the case) are addressed, if lesions are still present, depending on the presence of pruritus or other systemic signs, diseases such as contact allergy (for pruritic cases) or autoimmune disease can be considered (Fig. 7.1). Contact allergy is best ruled out by confinement, while autoimmune diseases require a skin biopsy of a primary lesion. As mentioned in Chapter 1 (this volume), superficial pyoderma is the most common complicating factor in the initial presentation.

Staphylococcal Folliculitis (Superficial Pyoderma)

Superficial pyoderma or bacterial folliculitis in horses is caused primarily by *Staphylococcus aureus*. Superficial pyoderma is one of the most common dermatological diseases in horses. Staphylococcal infections are secondary complicating diseases and should not be viewed as primary or idiopathic, as in the vast majority of cases there is a triggering cause. Therefore, clinicians should always strive to identify the underlying triggering disease to avoid repeated relapses of staphylococcal infections.

S. aureus is the same *Staphylococcus* sp. as that found in humans and is supposed to be present in low numbers as part of the normal flora. Infections are triggered when the number of *Staphylococcus* organisms increases (dysbiosis), misplacing other more benign bacteria that are part of the microbiome of the skin. The fact that the *Staphylococcus* sp. in horses and humans is the same is an important piece of information, as both horses and humans can temporarily carry the same bacteria if they are in contact with either other animals or other humans. If the *S. aureus* of the horse were to acquire methicillin resistance, humans in contact can become carriers of these resistant bacteria. This is relevant as carriage of MRSA in humans is difficult to eradicate and can predispose to MRSA infection if they have a wound or undergo surgery. Staphylococcal infection is not a contagious disease per se and, as mentioned before, these infections are always secondary to an underlying disease that

facilitates replication of the *Staphylococcus* that is already present on the skin. Thus, a horse with a staphylococcal infection is not a threat to another horse and will not cause an infection. However, horses that are in contact may temporarily carry the same strain as the one with the pyoderma and, if anything were to trigger an overgrowth of *Staphylococcus* in the second horse, this would be with the same strain as that of the stable mate. Thus, the strain that we carry on our skin may be important in the event that a *Staphylococcus* infection develops.

Staphylococcal pyoderma develops when an increased number of bacteria grow in the hair follicles. This abnormal replication leads to inflammation (folliculitis) and eventually to loss of the hair (alopecia). The first clinical signs of folliculitis are macules, papules and eventually pustules. The pustules are follicular (although this may not be easy to appreciate clinically) and, typically, are smaller than those of autoimmune diseases such as pemphigus. The pustules are transient, so the majority of patients present with crusting, scaling and hair loss (Fig. 7.2). The papules are responsible for the hair changing direction and giving the impression of hives (Fig. 7.3). Staphylococcal infections follow the pattern of distribution of the underlying disease. Sometimes, the lesions can appear more nodular in areas of trauma, as is the case with lesions in the saddle-pad areas (Fig. 7.4). In these cases, the bacteria are physically "pushed down" into the dermis, leading to more follicular damage. These lesions

Table 7.1. Differential diagnoses of crusting/scaling dermatitis.

Crusts due to pustular eruption		Crusts due to primary disease of keratinization
Follicular diseases	Non-follicular diseases	
Staphylococcal pyoderma	Dermatophilosis	Primary seborrhea
Dermatophytosis	Mites (e.g. *Chorioptes*)	
Dermodex infection	Allergies (e.g. insect, contact allergy)	
	Autoimmune disease (e.g. pemphigus foliaceus)	

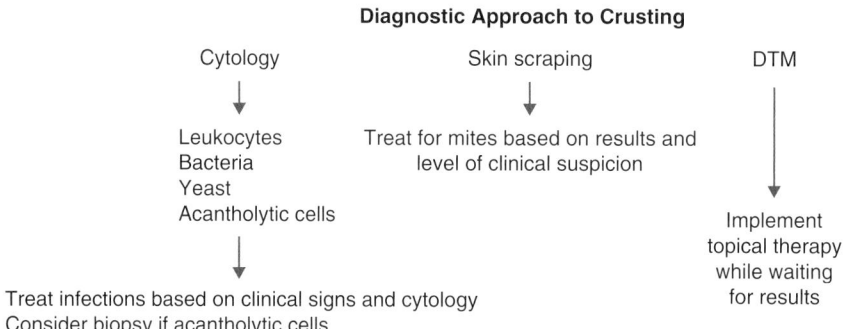

Diagnostic Approach to Crusting

Cytology → Leukocytes, Bacteria, Yeast, Acantholytic cells → Treat infections based on clinical signs and cytology. Consider biopsy if acantholytic cells

Skin scraping → Treat for mites based on results and level of clinical suspicion

DTM → Implement topical therapy while waiting for results

After ruling out mites, bacteria and fungi, consider skin biopsy to diagnose autoimmune disease or other less common diseases manifesting with crusting (e.g. sarcoidosis)

Fig. 7.1. Diagnostic approach to crusting dermatitis in horses. Cytology, skin scraping and fungal culture (DTM) comprise the basic testing to rule out most common causes (parasitic, bacterial and fungal infections).

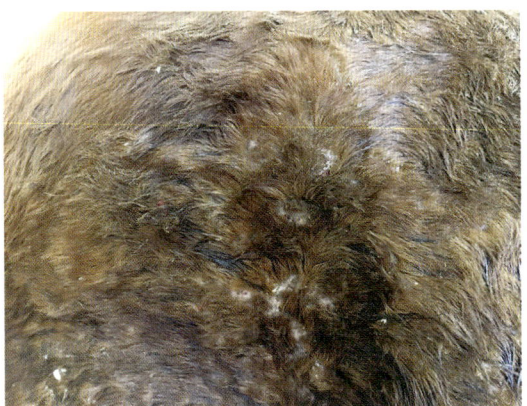

Fig. 7.2. Superficial pyoderma is a common cause of crusting in horses. As the pustules are transient, the most common presentation is crusting and epidermal collarettes, as visible in this young horse.

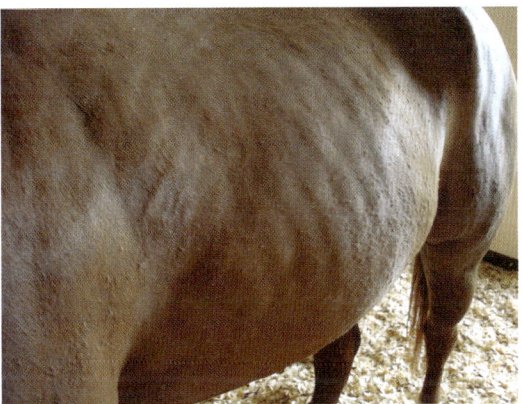

Fig. 7.3. A papular eruption of a superficial pyoderma may appear like hives from a distance, as shown in this horse diagnosed with bacterial folliculitis secondary to allergies.

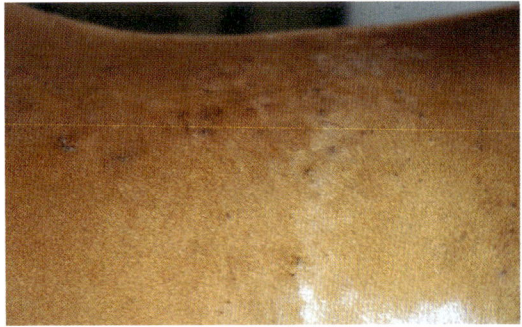

Fig. 7.4. Nodules can develop with pyoderma in areas of friction like the saddle pad of this horse diagnosed with a staphylococcal infection.

can be painful. It is important to remember that *Staphylococcus* is always present to some degree on the hair and in the hair follicles, so any practice that traumatizes the skin or hair, such as close skin clipping against the direction of hair growth, can trigger a bacterial folliculitis. Another manifestation of staphylococcal infection is the pyoderma that develops in most cases of pastern dermatitis. Pastern dermatitis is a syndrome of many causes, and the secondary infection aggravates the clinical picture, regardless of the underlying disease. Many horses with insect allergies are prone to "scratches," and cytology of the crusts reveals large numbers of cocci. A clinical presentation is crusting on the posterior

aspect of the pastern and fetlock region. Severe cases may be painful and lead to lower limb edema.

Diagnosis of staphylococcal pyoderma is largely a clinical diagnosis. Cytology can help when neutrophils and intracellular cocci are found. Sometimes, surface cytology is non-diagnostic as pustules are not present. Often, the diagnosis has to be clinical, based on the distribution and type of lesions.

Treatment can be topical or systemic. Topical therapy is always helpful as an adjunctive therapy, even in cases that are treated systemically. *Staphylococcus* traditionally is responsive to potentiated sulfonamides (25–30 mg/kg PO every 12–24 h for 2–4 weeks). As this antibiotic may trigger colitis, it is important to monitor horses for diarrhea or other signs of gastrointestinal distress. Very recently, at the University of Florida, several cases of resistant infections have been diagnosed. Therefore, if empirical treatment with sulfamethoxazole does not resolve the bacterial infection, it is strongly recommended that a sample is cultured from the patient to identify the correct antibiotic to use. If methicillin resistance is diagnosed in a horse, precautions should be taken by the personnel handling the patient to minimize the possibility of acquiring carriage of MRSA. Fluoroquinolones should be saved as far as possible for cases that truly require them to avoid the use of broad-spectrum antibiotics unless necessary. It is important to remember that this category of drug should not be used in growing animals due to the potential for cartilage damage.

Antimicrobial topical therapy can be done with benzoyl peroxide or chlorhexidine shampoos. Benzoyl peroxide is an excellent ingredient to kill bacteria; it removes the crusts and opens up the follicles. In people, it is frequently used for the treatment of acne due to these properties. Veterinary products have lower percentages of benzoyl peroxide than human products as an animal's skin is thinner and less greasy than human skin. Thus, it is important to use products that are designed for animals. One potential downside of benzoyl peroxide is its ability to dry the skin, which may be undesirable for chronic use. Therefore, if the skin is no longer crusty, it may be good either to add a moisturizing conditioner or to switch to an ingredient that causes less degreasing such as chlorhexidine. Regardless of the ingredient used, it is important to allow sufficient contact time (5–10 min) before rinsing. It is also important to be gentle during topical therapy with no aggressive scrubbing or plucking of the crusts to avoid pain and unnecessary scarring.

Some products may contain silver as an antimicrobial agent. For localized infections, sprays containing oxychlorine can be useful. Localized resistant infections may be treated with topical antibiotics. One good choice is mupirocin as it has a very good penetration and is effective in resistant cases.

The duration of treatment for pyoderma is very important. Most patients require treatment for pyoderma for a minimum of 2 weeks. It is important to remember that shorter antibiotic treatments and premature discontinuation of the antibiotic may predispose to relapses and eventually promote resistance due to suboptimal and repeated exposure of the bacteria to the antibiotic.

Dermatophytosis

Dermatophytosis (ringworm) is an overdiagnosed fungal disease in veterinary dermatology. Actual confirmed cases of dermatophytosis are not very common and are more likely to be seen in young, stressed animals or in geriatric horses with metabolic or endocrine diseases. Most of the cases that are clinically assumed to be fungal infections are actually bacterial infections. Thus, if it looks like ringworm, most of the time it is actually a bacterial folliculitis.

The most common dermatophytes affecting horses include *Trichophyton equinum*, *Trichophyton mentagrophytes*, *Trichophyton verrucosum*, *Microsporum gypseum* and *Microsporum canis*. *T. equinum* is the most common causative agent of dermatophytosis of horses. Two varieties of *T. equinum* have been reported, *T. equinum* var. *equinum* and *T. equinum* var. *autotrophicum*. *T. equinum* can be zoonotic, and transmission of infections from horses to riders

has been reported; therefore, care should be taken when handling infected horses.

It is important to know that exposure to dermatophytes does not always lead to establishment of infection. Some individuals appear to be more predisposed than others, possibly related to the type of immune response mounted by the individual. The outcome after exposure depends on the virulence of the dermatophyte, the condition of the skin, environmental conditions and the immune status of the host. Any damage to the skin barrier, due either to trauma or to excessive moisture, can predispose to the development of infection. Abrasions or microtrauma caused by insects or scratching can facilitate penetration of the dermatophyte. Allergic individuals are at increased risk of developing infection for a number of reasons. One is that they are itchy and traumatize their skin. Another is that they may be exposed more frequently to drugs such as glucocorticoids to decrease the itch and inflammation in their skin. Finally, they are prone to develop a humoral response (T-helper cell type 2 (Th2) response) rather than a cell-mediated (Th1) response. A humoral response is not protective against dermatophytes; instead, a cell-mediated response is required. Horses prone to a strong Th1 response are less likely to develop dermatophytosis in the first place, and if they do, they are quicker at recovering from it.

The development of cell-mediated immunity correlates with the development of an inflammatory response and is associated with clinical cure, whereas the lack of or a defective cell-mediated immunity predisposes the host to chronic or recurrent dermatophyte infection. The inflammatory reaction also promotes keratinocyte proliferation, which facilitates elimination of the fungus from the skin surface.

Dermatophytosis occurs more commonly in young horses. Stresses such as training, transportation or pregnancy increase the risk for developing the infection. Infections are more common in the winter in the north and in the summer in the south, in circumstances of overcrowding, poor sanitation and poor nutrition, and in places on the horse susceptible to microtrauma (e.g. by saddle or girth). Dermatophytes may be transmitted by contact with infected hairs from affected animals, asymptomatic carriers, the environment and fomites, tack (Figs 7.5 and 7.6), brushes, handlers or riders.

Clinical signs include patchy scaling and alopecia with or without inflammation and crusting, depending on the organism and the host response. Sometimes,

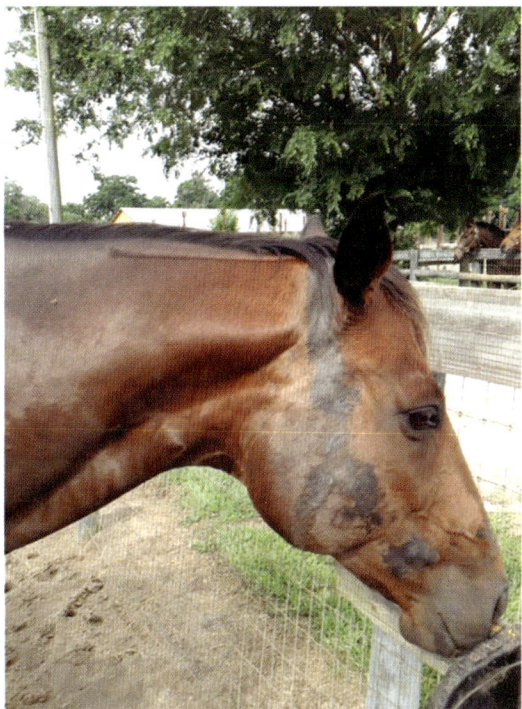

Fig. 7.5. Dermatophytosis transmitted by using an infected halter, as shown by the distribution of the alopecia.

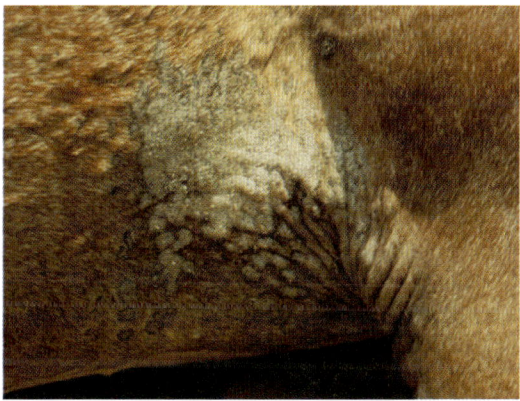

Fig. 7.6. Dermatophytosis in the girth area due to exposure to infected tack.

these may appear to be urticarial at initial onset, and may be either pruritic or non-pruritic. Differential diagnoses to consider with this presentation are superficial pyoderma/bacterial folliculitis, dermatophilosis, contact allergy, pemphigus foliaceus, occult sarcoid for localized lesions, hypersensitivity

and onchocerciasis. When cytology is done, it is not uncommon to find bacteria and neutrophils, as secondary bacterial infections are common. Some cases of dermatophytosis may cause acantholysis due to the severe exocytosis of neutrophils in the epidermis. The proteases released by the degenerating neutrophils can trigger acantholysis. Thus, the presence of acantholytic cells should not automatically be assumed to indicate pemphigus foliaceus, and fungal culture should be done in all cases where acantholytic cells are found. In older animals, mycosis fungoides should also be added to the list of differential diagnoses for patches of hair loss, scaling and crusting. In these cases, a biopsy is necessary to confirm the diagnosis.

Fungal culture is the most reliable diagnostic test for dermatophytosis and should be used in cases where bacterial folliculitis has been ruled out. The area should be treated with alcohol to decrease contamination by saprophytic fungi. After the alcohol has evaporated, hairs can be plucked, taking care that the roots are included. DTM is often used, although it has been demonstrated to be inferior to Sabouraud dextrose agar. It is important to note that *T. verrucosum* may not grow on DTM, and may require Sabouraud dextrose agar for a positive diagnosis. At the optimum incubation temperature of 27°C (80.6°F), a color change to red can be observed in the DTM only a few days after inoculation with infected hairs. The color change requires approximately 4 days for *T. equinum* and 5 days for *T. mentagrophytes*. It is important that the growth of the colony and the change of color of the medium occur at the same time for it to be a positive culture. Other fungi can induce a color change but typically take a longer time than that required by a dermatophyte. Once colony growth is observed, identification should be done to confirm the diagnosis and identify the source of infection. It is important to note that false-positive results with DTM can also occur. In specimens obtained from horses, a high contamination rate (36%), mostly from molds, was found with a cycloheximide-supplemented medium, making the examination of these cultures for the growth of dermatophytes impossible (Schmidt, 1996). For this reason, it is important to treat the area with alcohol before plucking hairs to submit for culture.

It is generally recommended that one or two drops of soluble B vitamin complex are added to the medium because some equine dermatophyte species will not grow without it. Other tests may indicate the presence of a dermatophyte infection but do not provide information about the genus or species. These include 10–20% KOH preparations or chlorphenolac preparations of plucked hairs to find ectothrix spores, as well as a biopsy and Wood's lamp examination.

Treatment for dermatophytosis is usually topical in conjunction with correction of the predisposing factors (e.g. crowding, poor nutrition, stress). Topical therapy can be done with a 2% chlorhexidine, 2% miconazole or 1% ketoconazole shampoo. After shampooing, a fungicidal dip solution can be used on the entire animal once daily for 7 days and then once weekly until resolution. It is important to remember that, even if the lesions are localized and focal, arthrospores may be present on the whole animal and thus treatment should not be limited to spot treatment of the individual lesions. This is an aspect of treatment that is frequently overlooked and may lead to treatment failure. Another consideration is that all animals in contact with the infected horse, whether they are symptomatic or not, should be considered potentially infected. Thus, it is recommended to either do cultures for all animals in contact or, minimally, to do an initial mild sulfur dip for all animals in contact to decrease the number of arthrospores present on their coat. In clinically affected horses, hair regrowth should not be used as an indication of cure because regrowth can occur while animals remain infected. It is therefore important to reculture a sample from the animal and demonstrate a lack of dermatophyte growth. Horses with low numbers of arthrospores on their coat may fluctuate between positive and negative cultures, so three consecutive negative cultures at 2-week intervals are recommended for confirmation.

The most effective topical options are 2% lime sulfur, 0.2% enilconazole (Imaverol; not approved for use in horses in USA at this time), natamycin 100 p.p.m. spray twice weekly (not approved in the USA at this time) and topical ketoconazole (e.g. Nizoral shampoo). No controlled studies have evaluated the efficacy of these products in equine dermatophytosis.

Dermatophytosis in otherwise healthy horses typically undergoes spontaneous remission within 3 months with topical therapy and environmental decontamination. It is important to discontinue training/working to promote healing. Continued trauma and exercise may exacerbate the infection and prolong recovery, especially in areas of contact with tack. It is good practice to keep the skin clean and dry

and to avoid prolonged contact with damp saddle pads and to wash pads frequently using bleach.

Systemic therapy is not usually recommended because of the expense, lack of proven efficacy, lack of knowledge regarding the pharmacokinetics of antifungals in horses and likelihood of spontaneous resolution. Although various dosages of griseofulvin have been recommended for the treatment of equine dermatophytosis, no published studies support this drug's efficacy and appropriate dose. Griseofulvin is teratogenic in horses, as it is in other species. The cost of azoles makes it challenging to use them for the treatment of dermatophytosis. This, combined with the spontaneous resolution in the majority of immunocompetent animals, leads to the rare recommendation of oral antifungal for dermatophytosis.

An integral aspect of management of dermatophytosis is to relieve overcrowding, correct any nutritional problems, separate affected horses from non-affected horses, handle "clean" horses before affected ones and treat the environment. Environmental treatment involves cleaning and treating relevant fomites, tack, brushes, combs and other equipment, cleaning the premises and treating the environment (e.g. stables, fences) with 5% lime sulfur, 5% sodium hypochlorite or 0.2% enilconazole. Vaccines have been used in the past in small and large animals to manage endemic dermatophytosis. Immunity obtained after vaccination appears to be cross-reactive. Currently, however, there are no commercially available vaccines for prevention of equine dermatophytosis in the USA.

In terms of public health considerations, all persons who may come in contact with affected animals or the infected hairs should be warned of the problem and instructed in appropriate preventative measures such as washing with an antifungal soap and wearing protective clothing that is then laundered. Infections in humans are typically self-limiting if the person is not immunocompromised.

Malassezia Dermatitis

Malassezia dermatitis is a secondary yeast infection that can occur particularly when the skin has been wet for extended periods of time, as in the case of fly masks that are left in place despite the occurrence of rain and sweat (Fig. 7.7). Many of these cases have secondary bacterial and yeast infections, both of which can contribute to pruritus. Crusting, alopecia and depigmentation are presentations of

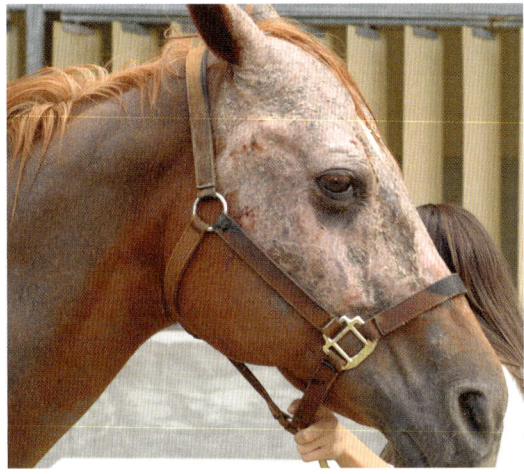

Fig. 7.7. *Malassezia* dermatitis on the face of a mare that had a fly mask left in place for weeks despite the occurrence of rain and sweat.

Malassezia dermatitis. Diagnosis is made by cytology. The exact number of yeast cells per high-power field necessary to make a diagnosis of *Malassezia* dermatitis is not known, as each patient is different. Thus, the results of the cytology need to be interpreted in the context of the clinical signs of the patient. Most cases of *Malassezia* dermatitis are treated topically and by correcting the predisposing cause. Shampoos that are effective at killing *Malassezia* contain 1–2% ketoconazole or 1% miconazole. Chlorhexidine can be used in cases where there are both bacterial and yeast infections.

Dermatophilosis

Dermatophilosis is a pustular and crusting bacterial disease in horses caused by *Dermatophilus* spp. This disease is also called streptothricosis, mycotic dermatitis, lumpy wool, strawberry foot rot, rain rot, rain scald, mud fever and dew poisoning. It is a relatively common disease that occurs throughout the world. It primarily affects horses, cattle, sheep and goats. It has recently been reported in dogs, cats and captive alligators in the southeastern USA, and is zoonotic.

Dermatophilus congolensis is a Gram-positive, non-acid-fast, aerobic or facultative anaerobic actinomycete. *Dermatophilus* has a distinct life cycle and exists in two morphological forms, hyphae and zoospores. *Dermatophilus* has been isolated from the soil, and its survival appears to depend on the type of soil and the water content. Because the

pathogenicity of *D. congolensis* seems to be preserved in soil, it is hypothesized that soil may act as a temporary reservoir for this organism. *Dermatophilus* can also survive in the skin of animals that are clinically normal, potentially acting as source of infection once favorable conditions become present. Crusts from affected animals represent an important source of contagion for spreading lesions on the same animal and possibly infection of other animals in the same herd. Chronically affected animals are the primary source of infection. However, they only become a serious source of infection when their lesions become wet, which results in the release of zoospores, the infective stage of the organism. Mechanical transmission of the disease occurs by both biting and non-biting flies. It can also be spread by contaminated clippers. Normal healthy skin is quite impervious to infection with *D. congolensis*. Predisposing factors that result in decreased resistance of the skin are necessary for infection to occur. Prolonged wetting of the skin by rain is one of the most important factors for increasing susceptibility to disease, and the first lesions often occur 2–3 weeks after the onset of the rainy season. Additional factors include microtrauma to the skin (e.g. insect bites and self-trauma due to allergic skin disease) or systemic illness/poor nutrition. The environment may be a source for recontamination because the zoospores resist drying at 100°C (212°F) and can survive in dry scabs at 28–31°C (82–88°F) for 42 months (Martinez and Prior, 1991). The immune response of the host is crucial in determining resistance to the development of the infection despite exposure to the organism, with a cell-mediated response being important to clear the infection.

The primary lesion of dermatophilosis is a papule, which progresses into a pustule and then into crusts and epidermal collarettes. The lesions easily become exudative, and hairs become matted together to form thick crusts in which the hairs are embedded. These crusts are tightly adherent to the skin and are painful when lifted. The skin underneath is frequently eroded. The lesions are not pruritic; instead, they are tender and the horse is reluctant to be touched. The exudate underneath is typically yellow-green. In this phase, cytology easily reveals the organism. The classic location of the lesions is dorsal (Fig. 7.8). When the infection becomes chronic, the lesions are dry and scaly (Fig. 7.9). The crusts are much thinner and the cytology is often negative. Frequently, the lesions are misdiagnosed as a fungal infection. Occasionally, the lesions are limited to the caudal aspect of the pastern region of the horse (Fig. 7.10) or the muzzle of foals (Fig. 7.11) when the mother is severely infected (Fig. 7.12). As *Dermatophilus* produces proteolytic enzymes, severe infections in foals may mimic autoimmune blistering diseases (Figs 7.13–7.15) Horses with white areas may develop severe erythema at these sites (Fig. 7.16); photosensitization has been

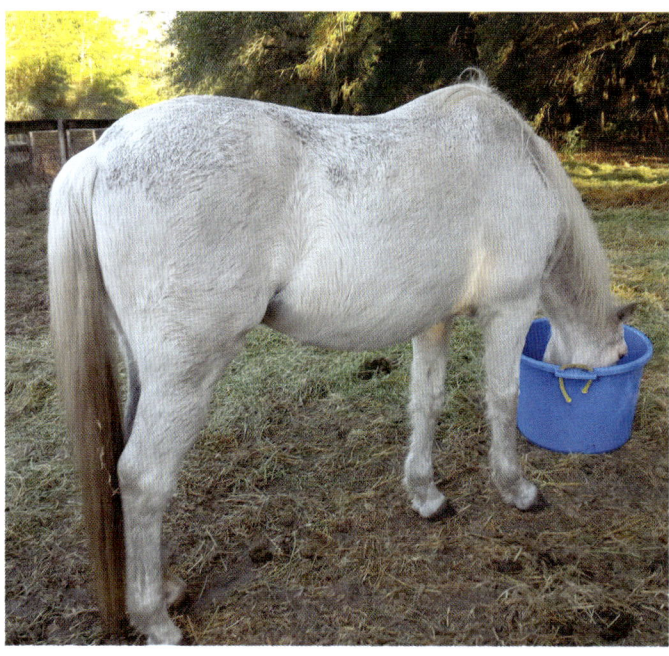

Fig. 7.8. Dermatophilosis on the dorsum of a geriatric horse. Note the distribution of the lesions that spare the ventral half of the body. In this case, thick crusts were tightly adherent to the body and were painful if lifted.

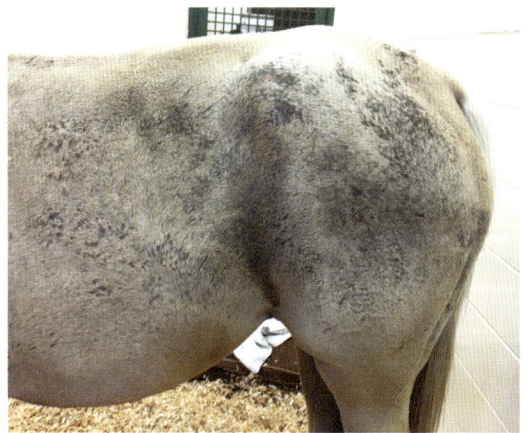

Fig. 7.9. Dry, chronic form of dermatophilosis. Note the paintbrush appearance of the lesions. This horse was also pruritic and had created some areas of self-trauma on his sides.

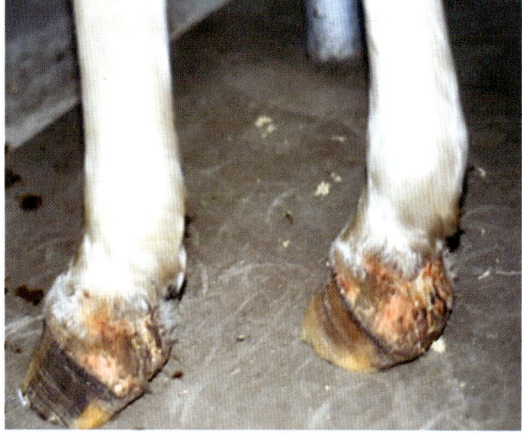

Fig. 7.10. Dermatophilosis on the pastern of a horse due to persistent exposure to moist grass. This form is also referred to as "grease heels" and is common in the summer time.

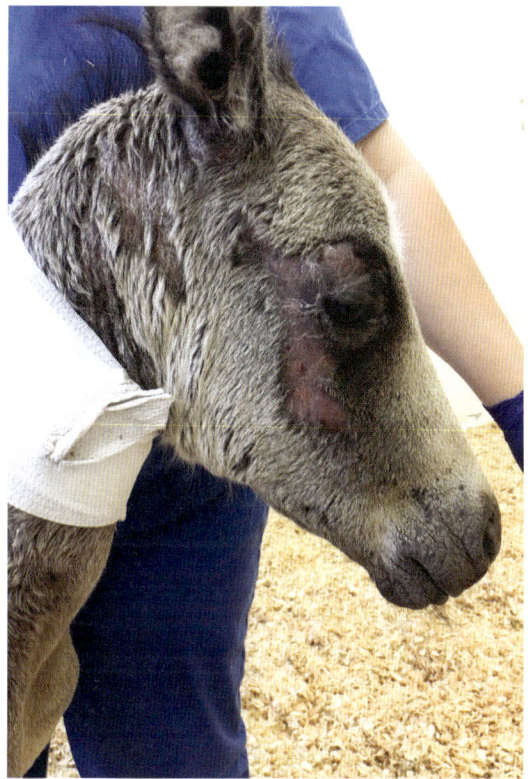

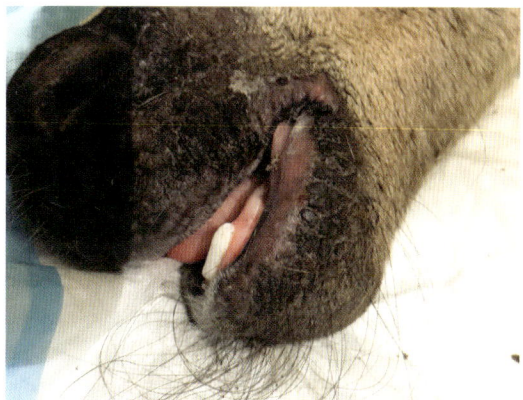

Fig. 7.13. Close-up of the muzzle of the foal shown in Fig. 7.11. Note the crusting and erosions. *Dermatophilus* can release proteolytic enzymes that can mimic the appearance of autoimmune diseases.

Fig. 7.11. A young foal with dermatophilosis on the face. Note the pustular eruption on the muzzle and the periocular hair loss.

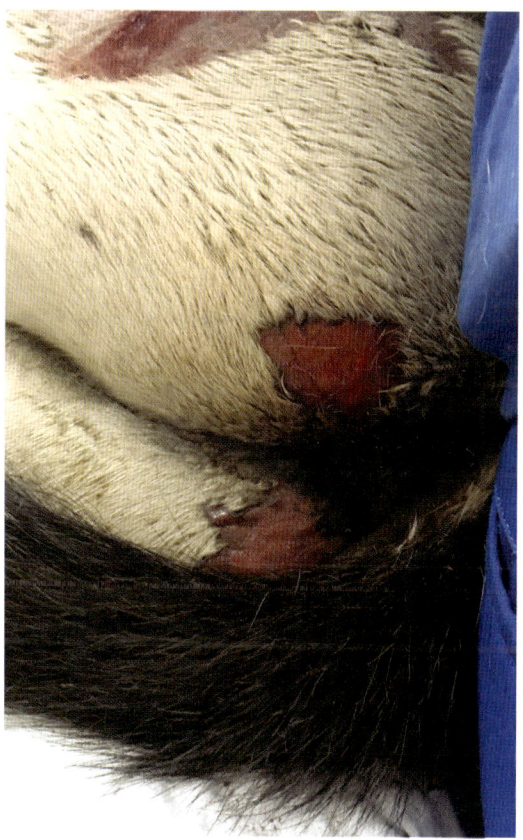

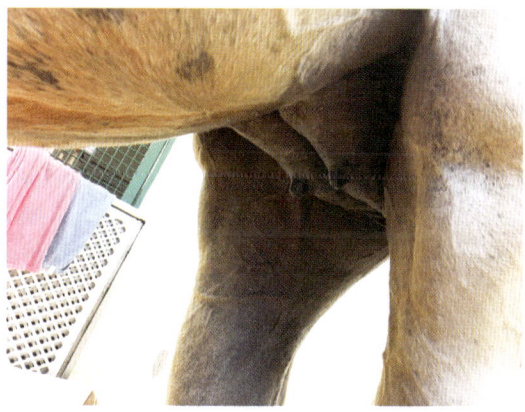

Fig. 7.12. Lesions on the groin of the mare who was the dam of the foal shown in Fig. 7.11. Note the crusting dermatitis and multifocal spotted alopecia.

Fig. 7.14. Ulcerative lesions on the perineal area of the foal shown in Fig. 7.11.

hypothesized to be involved in the pathogenesis of these lesions.

The clinical features of dermatophilosis are fairly characteristic but need to be confirmed by cytology.

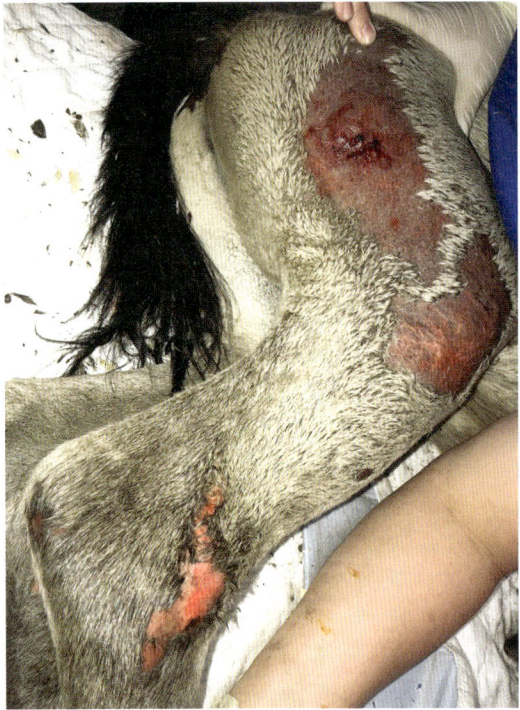

Fig. 7.15. Ulcerative lesions on pressure points of the foal shown in Fig. 7.11.

A "*Dermatophilus* prep" is the best way to look for this bacteria on cytology (Figs 7.17 and 7.18). This involves taking a portion of one of the crusts, mincing it with a scalpel blade and mixing it with a few drops of sterile water on a glass slide. The slide is then heated with a match until the saline has evaporated and stained with Diff-Quick, Gram stain or Giemsa stain. The slide is examined microscopically using a 100× oil-immersion lens. Touch impressions of the moist undersurface of the crust or the moist skin lesion may also be useful. *D. congolensis* is a branching, Gram-positive organism. The filaments can usually be seen dividing both transversely and longitudinally into thick bundles of coccoid forms creating the characteristic "train-track" appearance. Occasionally, it is necessary to culture the organism if the direct microscopic examination is either negative or questionable. This is best done with blood agar, resulting in rough, brown "applesauce drop" colonies. Recent studies have also investigated the polymerase chain reaction (PCR) for the diagnosis of *Dermatophilus* in cases that have negative cytology (García *et al.*, 2013; Frank *et al.*, 2016); this is a more sensitive methodology, although it may not be widely used in clinical settings.

Although most cases of dermatophilosis will spontaneously regress with the advent of dry weather, certain measures are beneficial. This disease will usually take 6–8 weeks to cure. Affected animals should be protected from further exposure to rainfall. Thorough (but gentle) grooming will remove many of the crusts and should be encouraged. Antimicrobial

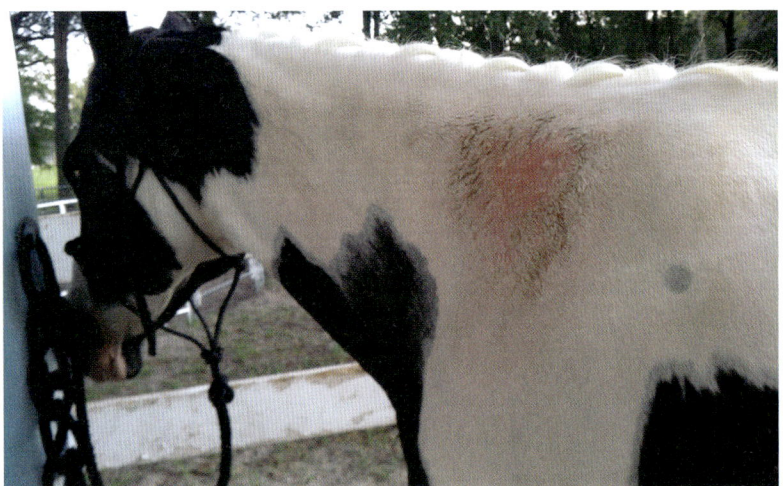

Fig. 7.16. Erythema due to photosensitization in a horse with localized dermatophilosis.

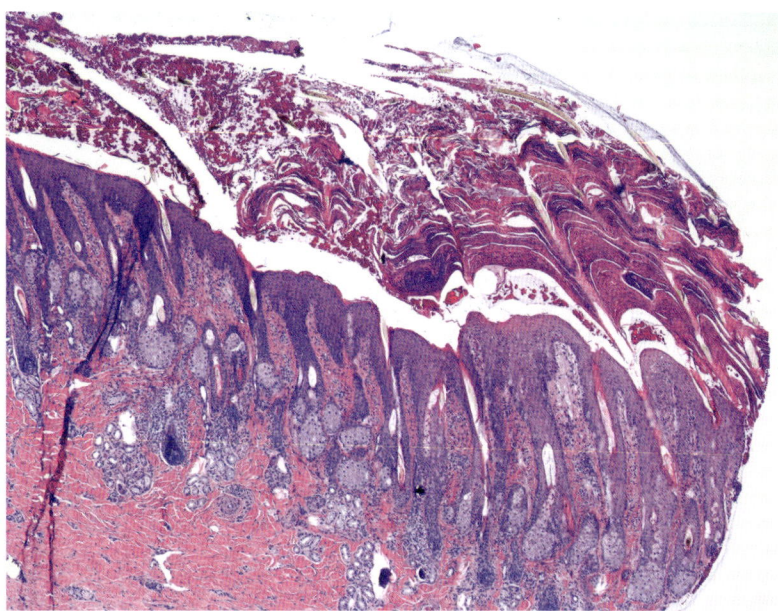

Fig. 7.17. Histopathology of a case of dermatophilosis. Note the thick multilayered crust that spans multiple hair follicles and the marked epidermal hyperplasia (40× magnification). (Image courtesy of Dr William Craft, University of Florida.)

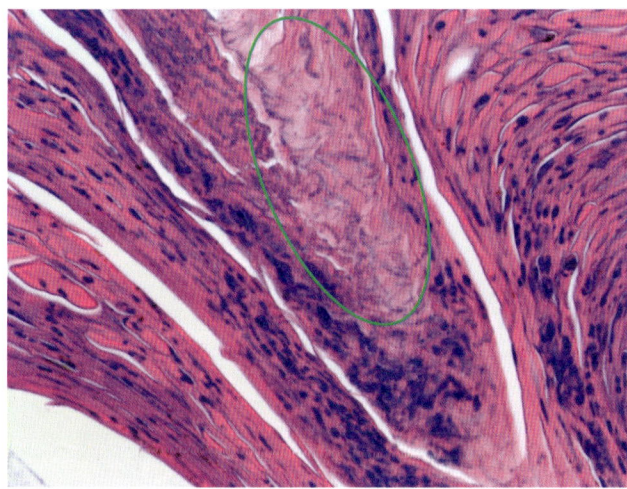

Fig. 7.18. Close-up of the biopsy sample shown in Fig. 7.17. The oval shape highlights the heavy presence of *Dermatophilus* in the crust (600× magnification). (Image courtesy of Dr William Craft, University of Florida.)

shampoo can be used to soften the crusts to promote removal. Benzoyl peroxide (2%) or chlorhexidine (2%) shampoos are effective. Shampoos should be used once or twice weekly allowing 10 min of contact, followed by thorough rinsing and drying.

Excessive scrubbing should be discouraged because it leads to trauma in the hair follicles and increases the risk of furunculosis. It is important not to share grooming tools between affected and non-affected horses to minimize spread of the organism. For localized lesions, topical mupirocin (e.g. Bactoderm), a drug with excellent antibacterial properties and skin penetration, may be used. Other topical options include 0.4% stannous fluoride (e.g. Mediquine) to be applied daily and oxychlorine spray (e.g. Vetericyn) to be used several times daily. Both products are rapidly bactericidal and constitute a valid alternative to the labor-intensive shampoo therapy. It is important to burn or properly dispose of crusts to prevent spread to other animals. Topical chloromycetin preparations have been recommended for pastern involvement in the horse. Systemic antibiotics can also be prescribed: procaine penicillin 22,000 IU/kg intramuscularly with or without streptomycin 11 mg/kg every 12 h for 14 days is effective, and trimethoprim-sulfamethoxazole 15–25 mg/kg PO every 12–24 h is effective in most cases.

The most effective method for prevention of equine dermatophilosis is to minimize exposure to excessive moisture and insects. Insect repellents (e.g. 2% permethrin) should be applied at least once daily in tropical climates where high humidity and rainfall are present. Topical antibacterial therapy with antibacterial shampoos (e.g. benzoyl peroxide) is also helpful to decrease the bacterial load on the skin.

It is important to note that dermatophilosis is zoonotic. In people, it can cause pitted keratolysis, painful or pruritic folliculitis and subcutaneous nodules. Immunosuppressed individuals may be more susceptible to disease. Care should therefore be taken when handling infected animals.

Pemphigus foliaceus

Pemphigus foliaceus is an autoimmune disease that results from autoantibodies forming against the proteins (e.g. desmogleins) responsible for holding the keratinocytes together in the epidermis. Pemphigus is a type II hypersensitivity reaction, in which binding of IgG with the desmoglein triggers a cytotoxic reaction. The result is a loss of cohesion among keratinocytes. These cells are called acantholytic cells and can be seen on both cytology and skin biopsies. The development of autoantibodies can be triggered by antigenic stimulation, and desmoglein may be an innocent bystander of an immune response that was directed at something else. Possible antigenic stimulations anecdotally reported to be responsible for pemphigus are vaccines, infections, allergies or drugs. In some horses, no antigenic stimulation can be identified and they are considered idiopathic cases. Of the cases reported in the literature, 60% have been seen in Appaloosa horses, so it is believed that there may be a genetic predilection, although Thoroughbreds and others are also affected.

In pemphigus foliaceus, which is the most common form of pemphigus in animals, the primary lesion is a subcorneal pustule. Pustules in pemphigus may span multiple follicles and are larger than those seen with follicular diseases. As pustules are fragile, patients usually present with crusting and scaling.

The disease typically begins on the face, head (Figs 7.19–7.21) and legs (Fig. 7.22), and spreads to the entire body (Figs 7.23 and 7.24); it may also affect the genitalia. Involvement of the face and the

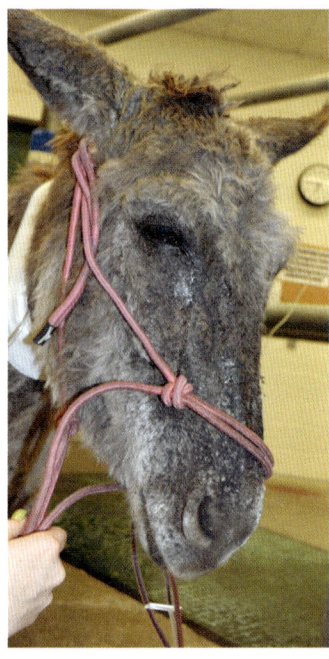

Fig. 7.19. Pustular eruption on the face of a donkey diagnosed with pemphigus foliaceus.

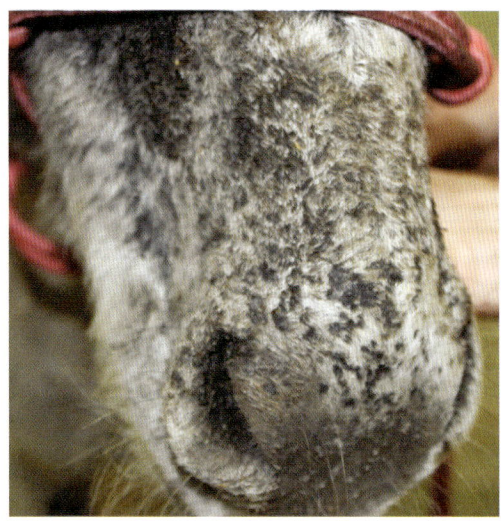

Fig. 7.20. Close-up of the dry pustules and crusts on the muzzle of the donkey shown in Fig. 7.19.

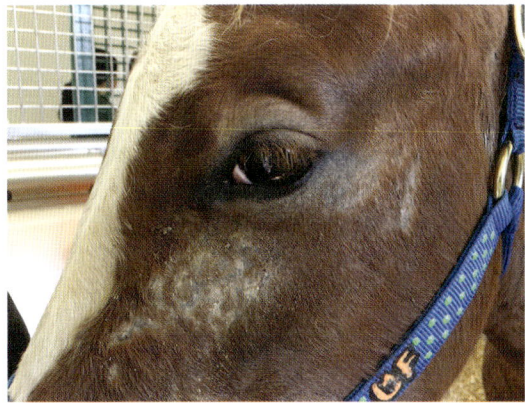

Fig. 7.21. Crusting and alopecia on the face of a young horse diagnosed with pemphigus foliaceus secondary to vaccination.

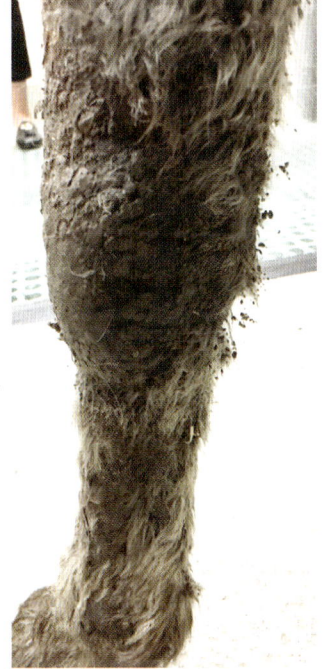

Fig. 7.22. Thick crusting and alopecia on the legs of a pemphigus foliaceus case.

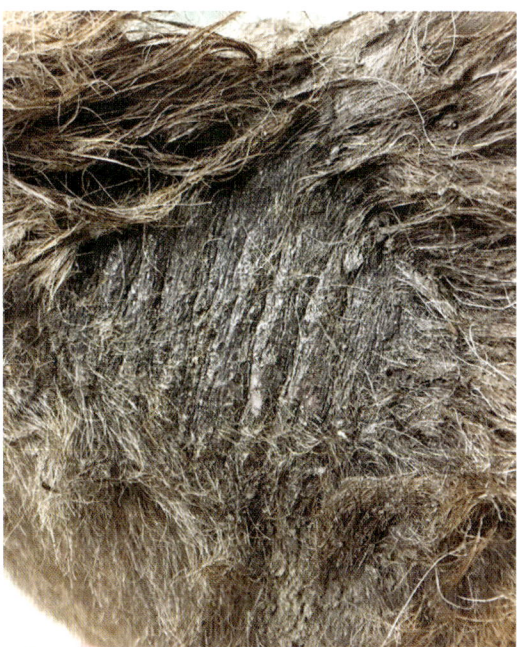

Fig. 7.23. Crusting dermatitis and alopecia on the neck of the patient shown in Fig. 7.22.

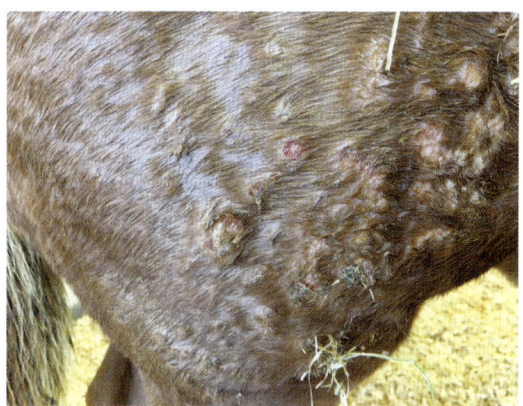

Fig. 7.24. Crusting and ulcerative lesions in a pemphigus foliaceus case believed to have been triggered by vaccination.

periocular area is a clue that this presentation, even when bacteria are present, is not a simple pyoderma. Lesions consist of alopecia, scaling and crusting; it is primarily an exfoliative disease. Sometimes, the pustular disease is confined to the coronary band (Figs 7.25 and 7.26). Other signs include depression,

limb edema, pyrexia and pruritus. The disease has a waxing and waning course. Many horses experience some form of depression and decreased appetite when they have a wave of lesions and may feel better once the lesions erupt.

In terms of age, there appear to be three different age groups. Most of the idiopathic cases seem to be

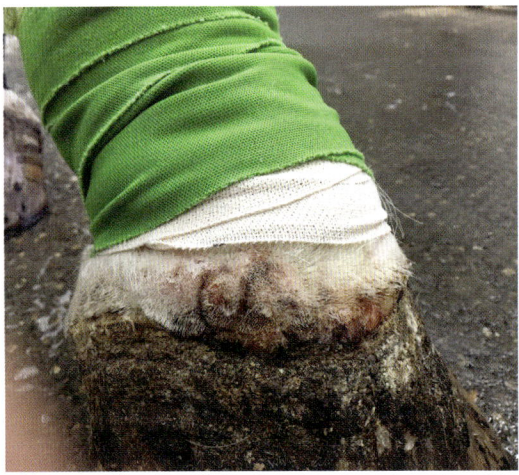

Fig. 7.25. Pustular eruption in a case of pemphigus foliaceus confined to the coronary band area.

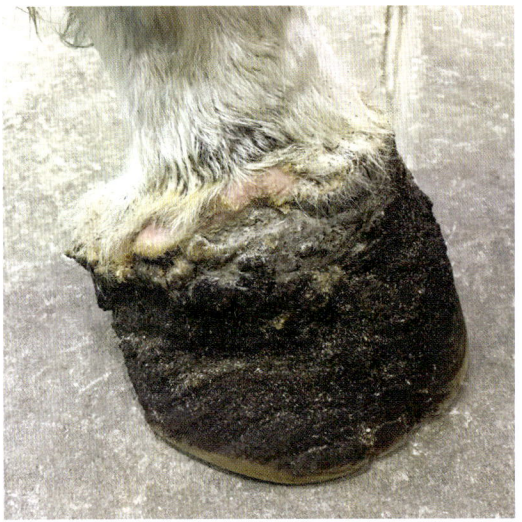

Fig. 7.26. A case of coronary band pemphigus.

middle-aged horses. Foals form another subset of pemphigus horses. These patients are believed to have reacted to an antigenic stimulation such as a vaccine (especially encephalitis vaccines or deworming). They tend to have a better prognosis than adult horses and often do not require long-term therapy. The final subset is older horses. These should be worked up for the presence of neoplasia, which may function as an antigenic trigger for the aberrant immune response leading to the attack on the skin.

The diagnosis of pemphigus is made based on clinical signs and supportive findings on cytology and skin biopsy. Cytology is the first step and often reveals acantholytic cells. It is important to remember that acantholytic cells may also occur with other diseases and do not always imply pemphigus. Any disease in which there is severe inflammation in the epidermis may lead to acantholysis, as proteases are released that can damage the desmogleins. It is therefore important to rule out these diseases (especially severe bacterial infection, contact allergy and dermatophytosis) before considering that the patient has pemphigus. A skin biopsy of an intact pustule for histopathology (subcorneal pustule with acantholytic cells) is essential. Histopathology shows pustules that span multiple follicles (Fig. 7.27). In subcorneal pustules, acantholytic cells appear as round cells that are larger than neutrophils. Figures 7.28 and 7.29 show examples of acantholytic cells.

Immunostaining can be done but is generally considered unnecessary. If no intact pustules are available, it is helpful to biopsy crusts; a good dermatopathologist can easily detect acantholytic cells within the crust. Many horses have a secondary infection at the time of the first visit, and the presence of severe pyoderma may mask the changes consistent with pemphigus. If possible, it is helpful to treat the secondary infection first, before taking a biopsy. Drugs can also interfere with the characteristic features of pemphigus. Therefore, it is important not to start glucocorticoid therapy until the biopsy has been taken.

Treatment for pemphigus involves identification of the triggering cause, if possible. As well as future avoidance of the trigger, immunosuppressive therapy may be needed to stop the aberrant immune response. Immunosuppressive therapy is needed in all cases in which a trigger cannot be identified (idiopathic pemphigus). Drugs or vaccines given in the 2 months prior to development of the lesions should be considered as a possible trigger, even if they have been given in the past without problem.

Treatment is with prednisolone 1.5–2.5 mg/kg PO once daily to start, with slow reduction (over several weeks) to a regimen of every other day. If no response is obtained with prednisolone, dexamethasone (0.02–0.1 mg/kg once daily) can be used for induction. Generally, the maintenance dose is 25% of the induction dose and is given every other day. Horses should be carefully monitored for the development of laminitis. The use of steroid-sparing agents is necessary in most cases to minimize the adverse effects of glucocorticoid therapy.

Azathioprine 2 mg/kg every other day has also been used successfully and allows the clinician to

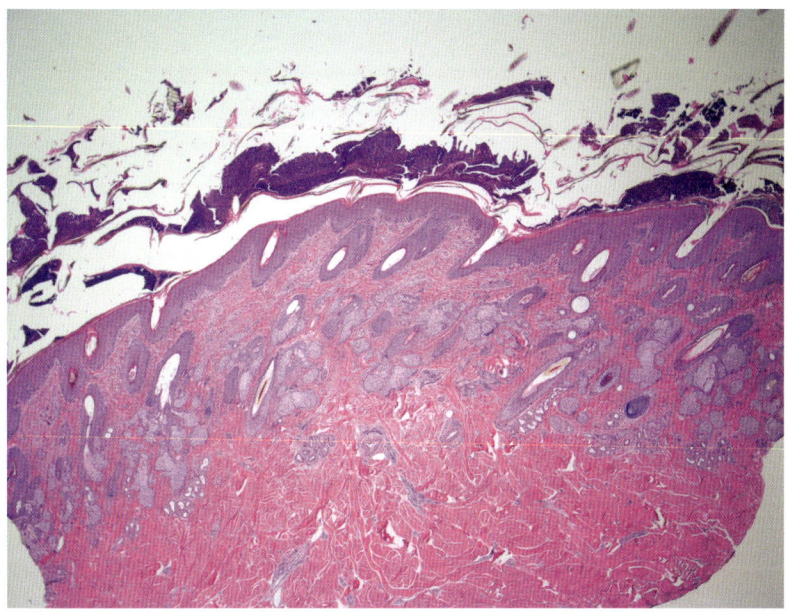

Fig. 7.27. Histopathology of pemphigus foliaceus. Note the pustular eruption that spans multiple follicles (20× magnification). (Courtesy of Dr William Craft, University of Florida.)

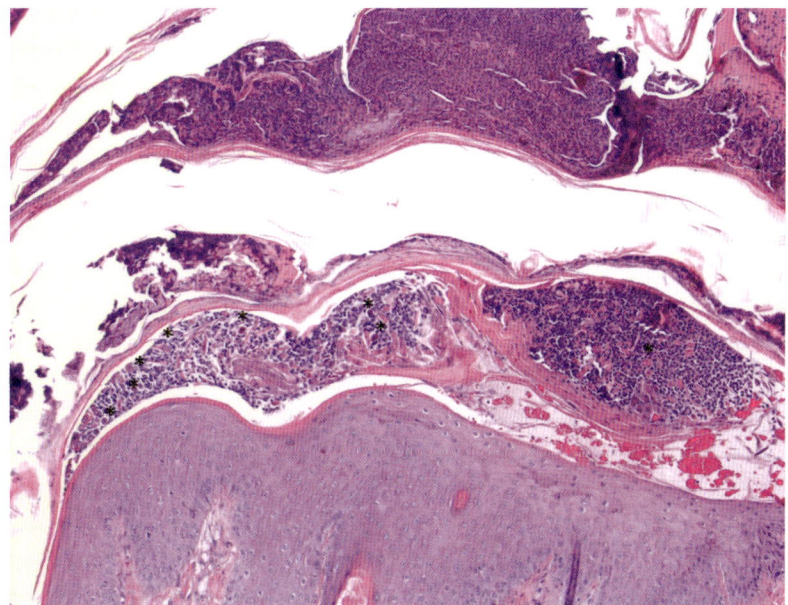

Fig. 7.28. Numerous acantholytic cells (round cells identified by asterisks; 100× magnification) evident in subcorneal pustule. (Courtesy of Dr William Craft, University of Florida.)

use a lower dosage of prednisolone. The bioavailability of azathioprine in horses is low, ranging from 1% to 7%, which may account for the poor response in some patients. Overall, this medication is well tolerated in horses, but it can be cost-prohibitive in the long term.

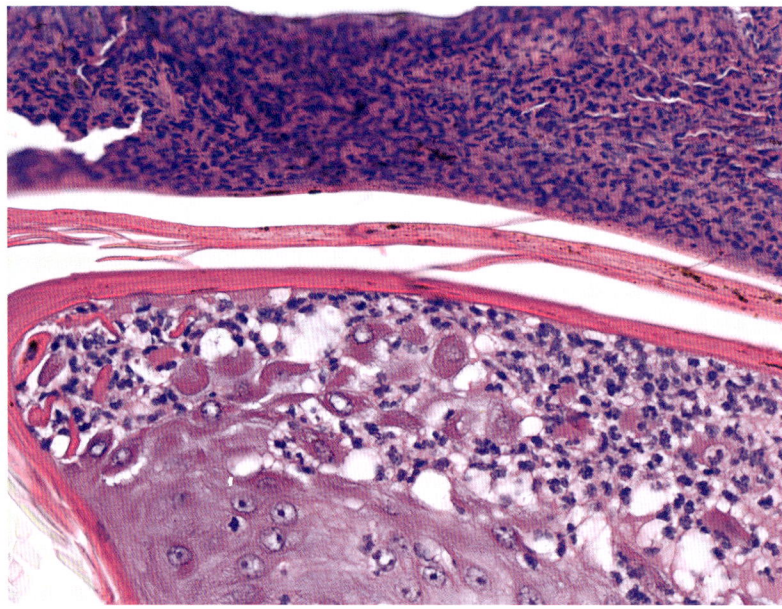

Fig. 7.29. An area of active acantholysis. Note the keratinocytes that are detaching and floating as round pink cells. At the top, note the thick crust with degenerated neutrophils (400× magnification). (Courtesy of Dr William Craft, University of Florida.)

The side effects of azathioprine include colic, secondary infections, hepatopathy and bone marrow suppression. A complete blood count and chemistry panel should be done prior to initiating therapy and repeated during treatment every 2 weeks for 6 weeks, and then every 4–8 weeks, depending on the horse's response. When the disease is in remission, the frequency of administration can be decreased to every 2–4 weeks. This therapy is less commonly used because of the potential for serious adverse side effects such as anemia, thrombocytopenia, leukopenia, proteinuria, hepatopathies and skin rashes. Ideally, a complete blood count, chemistry and urinalysis should be performed weekly; if economics is a consideration, at least a packed cell volume and urine dipstick test should be run. In young animals (foals), it has been found that treatment can be stopped after several weeks; adults usually require treatment for life.

Less Common Causes of Generalized Crusting in Horses

Some diseases in horses are systemic diseases that can also have cutaneous manifestations. Equine multisystemic eosinophilic epitheliotropic disease and generalized granulomatous syndrome are examples of this category.

Equine multisystemic eosinophilic epitheliotropic disease

This is a rare infiltrative eosinophilic disease that affects multiple body systems, including the gastrointestinal tract, abdominal organs, skin and occasionally the lungs. These horses present with crusting alopecia and pruritus (Figs 7.30–7.32) in conjunction with systemic signs such as weight loss, despite proper feeding, and sometimes in the absence of diarrhea, fever and lethargy. The dermatological work-up of these cases requires ruling out severe allergies including food allergies, parasites, infections and neoplastic diseases, in conjunction with the work-up of the other systemic signs associated with the specific case. Skin biopsy reveals massive infiltration with eosinophils in both the dermis and the epidermis (Figs 7.33 and 7.34). Glucocorticoid therapy can be attempted although the response is typically unsatisfactory. Prognosis is guarded to poor, and most horses are euthanized due to the progressive nature of this condition and the poor quality of life.

Idiopathic generalized granulomatous syndrome (equine sarcoidosis)

This is a rare condition in horses. It is believed to be the result of an excessive immune response against an

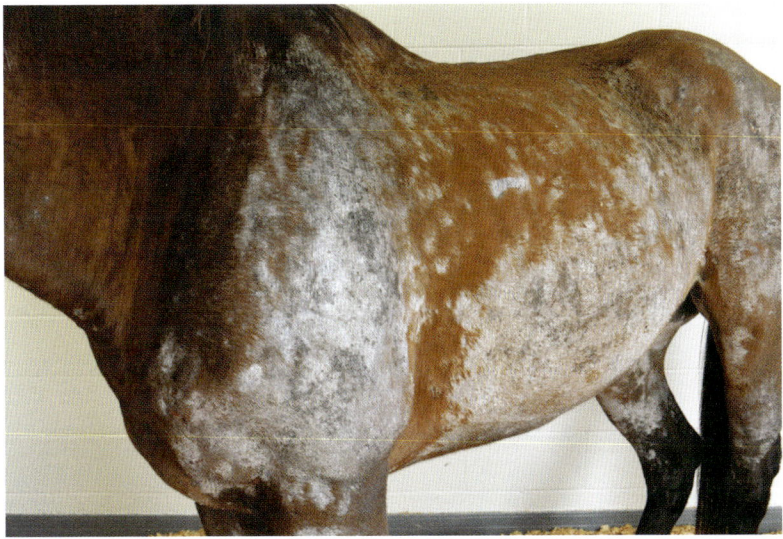

Fig. 7.30. A severe case of multisystemic eosinophilic epitheliotropic disease. In this patient, generalized crusting and hair loss was accompanied by weight loss.

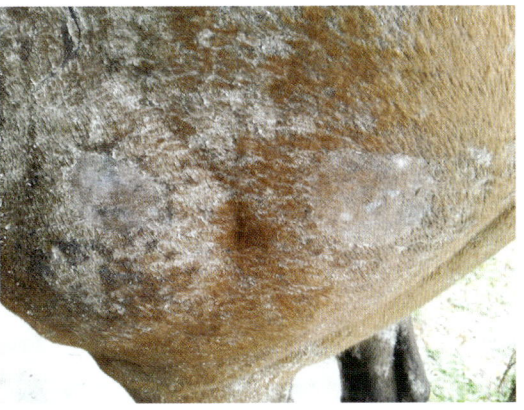

Fig. 7.31. Close-up of the patient shown in Fig. 7.30. Note the dry, almost exfoliative aspect of the lesions and the areas of alopecia.

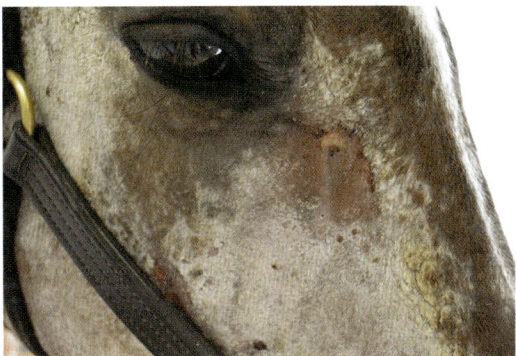

Fig. 7.32. Thick crusts mixed with silvery scaling and alopecia on the face of the patient shown in Fig. 7.30.

unidentified antigenic stimulation. Papillomavirus has been considered as a possible trigger, but efforts to identify this virus in the tissue have failed so far. The disease manifests as crusting and exfoliative dermatitis (Figs 7.35 and 7.36), wasting and granulomatous infiltration of internal organs. Pruritus is not usually a characteristic of sarcoidosis in horses. The lungs and gastrointestinal tract are the most frequently affected internal organs. Clinically, two main forms are described. One is characterized by crusting and alopecia, while the second, which is more rare, is nodular. Horses affected by the nodular form can also have crusting and alopecia. Many of these horses have poor appetite, weight loss and a history of colic.

Diagnosis is based on exclusion of other common cutaneous diseases manifesting with crusting and by histopathology of the skin. Biopsy reveals extensive infiltration of lymphocytes, histiocytes and multinucleated giant cells. It is important that samples are also submitted for culture to rule out infectious causes for the granulomatous inflammation.

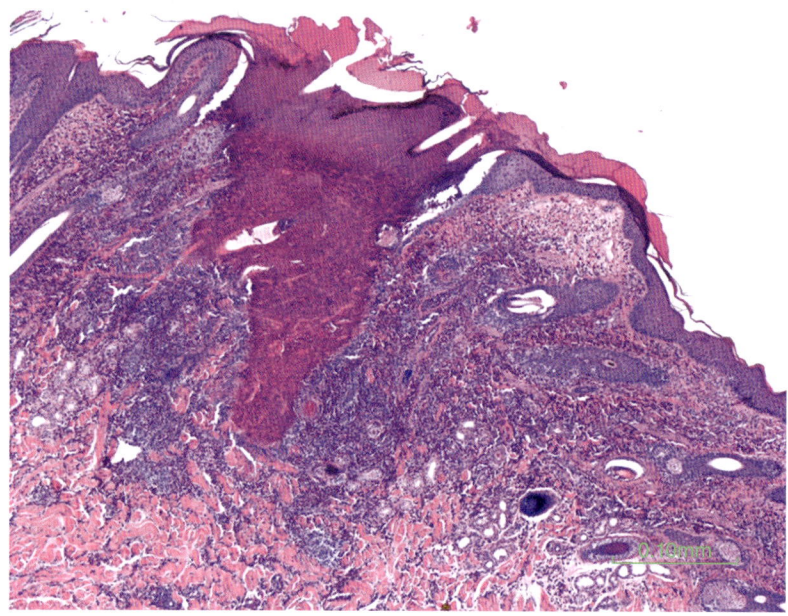

Fig. 7.33. Histopathology of a lesion from the patient shown in Fig. 7.30. Note the severe eosinophilic infiltrate that obliterates the epidermis in the area of ulceration. Inflammation is both superficial and deep (100× magnification). (Courtesy of Dr William Craft, University of Florida.)

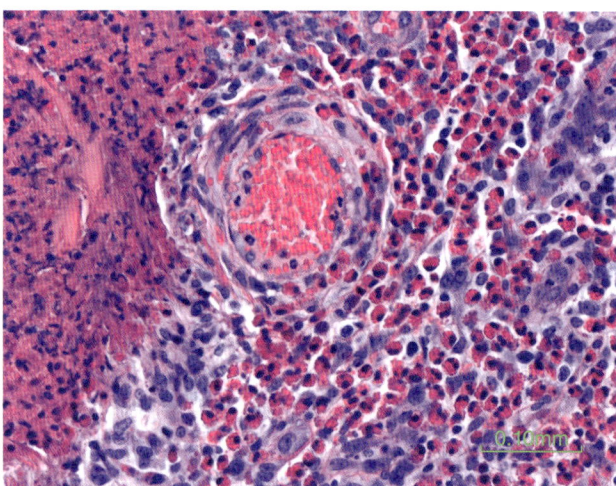

Fig. 7.34. Close-up of the lesion shown in Fig. 7.33, showing massive infiltration of eosinophils (400× magnification). (Courtesy of Dr William Craft, University of Florida.)

Treatment involves the use of glucocorticoids. A common choice is prednisolone at an initial dose of 1–2 mg/kg PO once daily (for 10–14 days), followed by a lower dose of 0.25–1 mg/kg PO once daily for several weeks. Most horses show a positive response, although some may be refractory to treatment. Even if a positive response is seen, treatment generally needs to be continued long term as relapses may occur if therapy is discontinued.

The prognosis for the generalized systemic disease is poor as the disease is progressive. Horses with localized disease typically have a better prognosis, and the disease may stay localized for a long time.

Occult sarcoids

Areas of localized crusting can be indication of an occult sarcoid. This form of sarcoid (Fig. 7.37) can

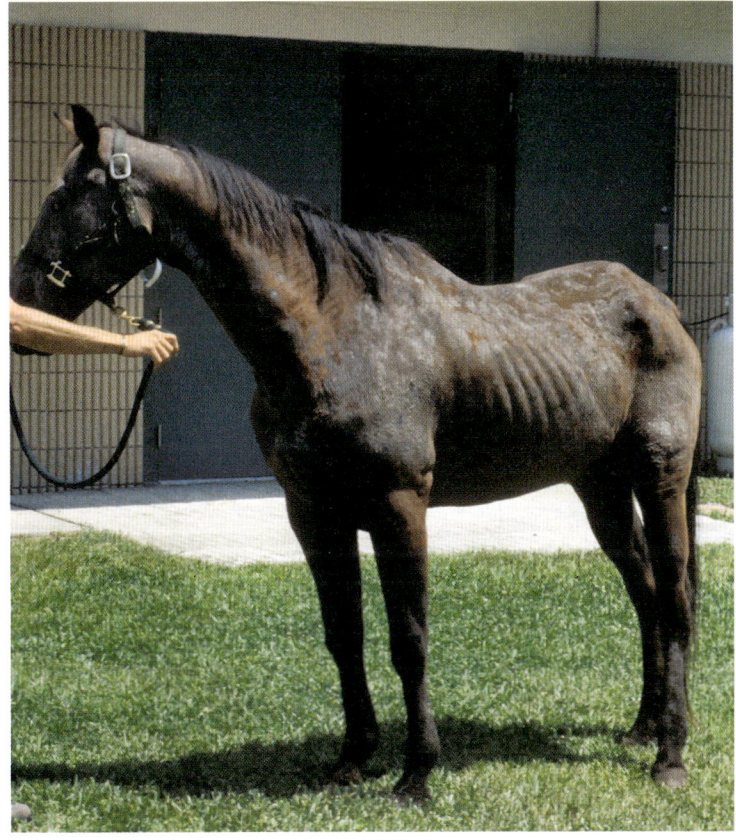

Fig. 7.35. Sarcoidosis associated with weight loss in a 10-year-old horse.

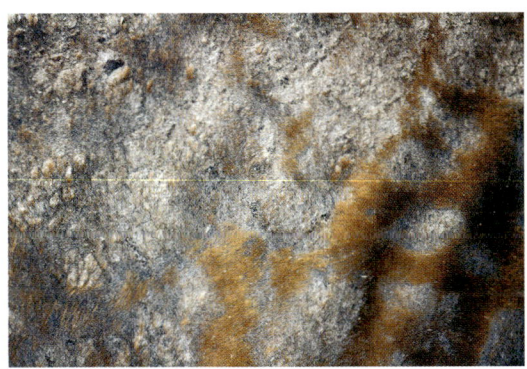

Fig. 7.36. Close-up of the lesions from the patient shown in Fig. 7.35, showing the crusting and patchy hair loss.

be confused with a localized infection of dermatophytes or superficial pyoderma. It can present with crusting and alopecia and may stay unchanged for a long time. This is when the history is very important, as well as the basic diagnostics to rule out infectious diseases that should be treated. As sarcoids can worsen with trauma, biopsy is often not recommended to avoid precipitating the behavior of the sarcoid.

Sebaceous adenitis

Sebaceous adenitis is a disease that is reported more frequently in dogs and presents with crusting and scaling. One report of sebaceous adenitis has been published in a horse (Osborne, 2006). This horse presented with progressive patches of non-pruritic scaling, crusting, alopecia and leukoderma. The diagnosis of sebaceous adenitis was made by histopathology, and spontaneous regression was reported concurrently with the regression of a sarcoid. Although this condition is rare, it is important to consider that a biopsy may be needed

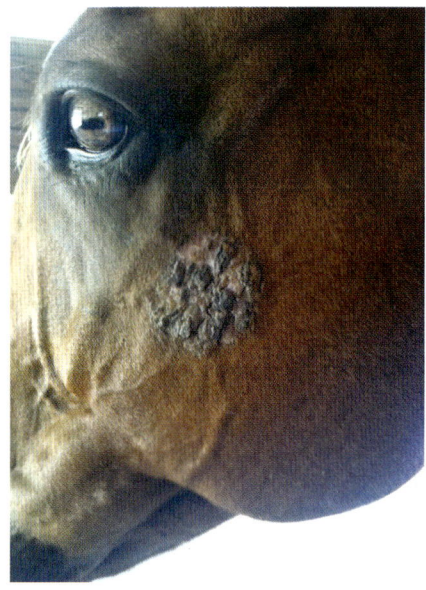

Fig. 7.37. Occult sarcoid on the face of a horse. This lesion was reported to have been present for over 2 years, largely unchanged.

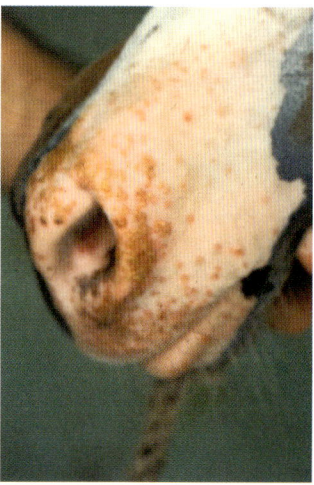

Fig. 7.38. Pustular eruptions caused by vesicular stomatitis virus infection. As well as pustules on the muzzle, ulcerative lesions were present in the oral cavity of this patient.

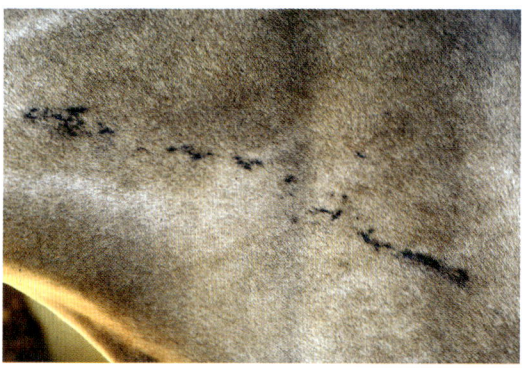

Fig. 7.39. Linear keratosis on the lateral neck of a horse.

if crusting is progressive and otherwise not consistent with more common diseases.

Viral diseases

Viral diseases of horses affecting the skin are rare in the USA. The most common is vesicular stomatitis virus. In this disease, pustules and crusts can be seen on the muzzle (Fig. 7.38). This virus is transmitted by biting insects such as *Culicoides* and also causes oral ulcerations with excessive salivation and ulcerations on the coronary band. Healing occurs naturally in 2 weeks.

Primary diseases of keratinization

As mentioned earlier, primary seborrhea is rare in the horse. One form of localized primary defect of keratinization is linear keratosis (Fig. 7.39). This is believed to be a genetically inherited disease, as it occurs more frequently in Quarter Horses. Lesions may be seen early in life as unilateral linear bands of hyperkeratosis and alopecia. The horse is otherwise healthy and not bothered by the lesions. This disease does not require treatment and does not spontaneously resolve. Topical keratolytic products can be used to aid in the removal of excessive crusting or to keep the crusts supple. Topical urea or propylene glycol mixed with water has been used to soften the lesions.

Cannon keratosis is another rare primary disease of keratinization. In this condition, crusting is present on the cranial aspect of the rear cannon bone areas. It is important that the work-up of these cases includes the more common causes of crusting, such as bacterial infections, insect allergies and contact allergy. Typically, affected horses are not pruritic, and this can help to discriminate from other conditions that usually have some form of pruritus. If the disease is truly a primary disease of keratinization, it persists for life unchanged; topical keratolytic therapy can be carried out to minimize the appearance of the crusts.

Summary and Diagnostic Approaches

Based on the information presented in this chapter, when approaching a case of crusting dermatitis it is important to consider the most common causes first (Table 7.1). Staphylococcal folliculitis is by far the most common disease and can be secondary to almost any underlying disease in dermatology. Staphylococcal infections secondary to allergic disease are statistically the most common cause for crusting dermatitis. Bacterial infections are confirmed by cytology. As bacteria complicate the vast majority of dermatological cases and at times mask recognition of the underlying disease, it is important to address these infections first and then re-evaluate.

Dermatophytosis can be seen in immunocompromised horses that are exposed to rain and have some skin trauma, which facilitates the establishment of infection by zoospores present in the environment. In the first evaluation, it is helpful to carry out cytology and evaluate the type of inflammatory infiltrate and the presence of bacteria. If the patient is pruritic, a skin scraping to look for mites is also indicated, particularly if the crusting affects the legs, as *Chorioptes* frequently affects the lower legs causing crusting and pruritus. Although dermatophytosis is uncommon in immunocompetent adult horses, it is good practice in the initial assessment to carry out cytology and a fungal culture by plucking hairs and culturing them on DTM in all cases of crusting disease.

When ranking the various differential diagnoses, it is important to highlight how the distribution of lesions is different in the various conditions. Staphylococcal folliculitis is typically a truncal disease and may superimpose dermatophilosis on the dorsum in tropical climates, while dermatophytosis may occur in other areas such as the girth or face, depending on how the infection occurred. Early cases of staphylococcal pyoderma may look like urticaria, while more advanced cases will have crusting, erosions and alopecia. In cases of dermatophytosis, the alopecia spreads toward the periphery, while the staphylococcal infection typically presents with smaller multifocal areas of raised hair (which clients may misrepresent as hives) and smaller patches of hair loss. It is important to note that dermatophytosis can be complicated by a secondary bacterial infection, and thus the detection of bacteria on cytology does not rule out the possibility that another cause of folliculitis is present in the same case.

For autoimmune causes of pustules such as pemphigus foliaceus, lesions typically present on the face and ears or on the coronary band area. Many patients have a history of loss of appetite or malaise when the wave of lesions occurs. The disease has a waxing and waning course, and occurs most frequently in middle-aged horses. Sometimes, pemphigus may be caused by vaccinations or drugs, rather than being idiopathic. Therefore, if very young patients are diagnosed with pemphigus, it is useful to have a detailed history of medications or vaccines given in the 3–6 weeks prior to development of the disease. Many of these cases have good prognosis as long as the trigger is identified and avoided in the future. Occasionally, these patients still require immunosuppressive therapy for a long time, even if there is no further exposure to the trigger. Immunosuppressive treatment is most commonly with a combination of glucocorticoids and azathioprine. Diagnosis of pemphigus is by biopsy. It is important to stress that acantholytic cells are sometimes seen with other diseases such as contact allergy or bacterial infection and thus it is important to address any infections before biopsy.

If the crusting primarily affects the legs, *Chorioptes* needs to be considered, and horses should be scraped to look for the mites. Horses with feathers are prone to *Chorioptes* infestation. Treatment for mites can be done topically with lime sulfur dips or fipronil spray, and by systemic administration of ivermectin. It is important to note that oral ivermectin may not always be effective as the mites are superficial, and therefore topical therapy is always recommended. All horses in contact with the infected horse need to be treated to avoid reinfestation. This needs to be done regardless of whether they are symptomatic or not.

Conclusions and Take Home Messages

Crusting can be caused by a variety of diseases. It is important to find out whether the disease is progressive and where it started on the body. The distribution of lesions and the presence of pruritus or systemic illness also need to be noted to help with the ranking of differential diagnoses. Cytology, skin scrapings and culture using DTM should be done in all cases as good practice. Once infections are treated and mites and dermatophytes have been ruled out, a biopsy should be considered to diagnose autoimmune disease or other less common diseases such as equine sarcoidosis.

References

Frank, L.A., Kania, S.A. and Weyant, E. (2016) RT-qPCR for the diagnosis of dermatophilosis in horses. *Veterinary Dermatology* 27, 431-e112.

García, A., Martínez, R., Benitez-Medina, J.M., Risco, D., Garcia, W.L. *et al.* (2013) Development of a real-time SYBR Green PCR assay for the rapid detection of *Dermatophilus congolensis*. *Journal of Veterinary Science* 14, 491–494.

Martinez, D. and Prior, P. (1991) Survival of *Dermatophilus congolensis* in tropical clay soils submitted to different water potentials. *Veterinary Microbiology* 29, 135–145.

Osborne, C. (2006) Sebaceous adenitis in a 7-year-old Arabian gelding. *Canadian Veterinary Journal* 47, 583–586.

Schmidt, A. (1996) Diagnostic results in animal dermatophytoses. *Zentralblatt für Veterinarmedizin Reihe B* 43, 539–543.

Further Reading

Staphylococcal pyoderma

Axon, J.E., Carrick, J.B., Barton, M.D., Collins, N.M., Russell, C.M. *et al.* (2011) Methicillin-resistant *Staphylococcus aureus* in a population of horses in Australia. *Australian Veterinary Journal* 89, 221–225.

Islam, M.Z., Espinosa-Gongora, C., Damborg, P., Sieber, R.N., Munk, R. *et al.* (2017) Horses in Denmark are a reservoir of diverse clones of methicillin-resistant and -susceptible *Staphylococcus aureus*. *Frontiers in Microbiology* 8, 543.

Parisi, A., Caruso, M., Normanno, G., Latorre, L., Miccolupo, A. *et al.* (2017) High occurrence of methicillin-resistant *Staphylococcus aureus* in horses at slaughterhouses compared with those for recreational activities: a professional and food safety concern? *Foodborne Pathogens and Disease* 14, 735–741.

Sloet van Oldruitenborgh-Oosterbaan, M.M., Troelstra, A., Barneveld, A., Wagenaar, J.A., Houwers, D.J. and van Duijkeren, E. (2008) Methicillin resistance *Staphylococcus aureus* in the horse clinic. *Tijdschrift Voor Diergeneeskunde* 133, 1056–1060.

Dermatophytosis

Abdel-Halim, M.M. and Kubesy, A.A. (1993) Evaluation of dermatophyte test medium for diagnosis of dermatophytosis among farm animals. *Journal of the Egyptian Veterinary Medical Association* 53, 207–210.

Cabanes, F.J., Abarca, M.L. and Bragulat, M.R. (1997) Dermatophytes isolated from domestic animals in Barcelona, Spain. *Mycopathologia* 137, 107–113.

Dahl, M.V. (1994) Dermatophytosis and the immune response. *Journal of the American Academy of Dermatology* 31, S34–S41.

Mahmoud, A.L. (1995) Dermatophytes and other keratinophilic fungi causing ringworm of horses. *Folia Microbiologica* 40, 293–296.

Ogawa, H., Summerbell, R.C., Clemons, K.V., Koga, T., Ran, Y.P. *et al.* (1998) Dermatophytes and host defense in cutaneous mycoses. *Medical Mycology* 36, 166–173.

Schutte, J.G. and van den Ingh, T.S. (1997) Microphthalmia, brachygnathia superior, and palatocheiloschisis in a foal associated with griseofulvin administration to the mare during early pregnancy. *Veterinary Quarterly* 19, 58–60.

Singh, K.V. and Agrawal, S.C. (1982) Nutritional requirements of keratinophilic fungi and dermatophytes for conidial germination. *Mycopathologia* 80, 27–32.

Veraldi, S., Genovese, G. and Peano, A. (2018) Tinea corporis caused by *Trichophyton equinum* in a rider and review of the literature. *Infection* 46, 135–137.

Wagner, D.K. and Sohnle, P.G. (1995) Cutaneous defenses against dermatophytes and yeasts. *Clinical Microbiology Reviews* 8, 317–335.

Dermatophilosis

Ambrose, N.C., Mijinyawa, M.S. and Hermoso de Mendoza, J. (1998) Preliminary characterisation of extracellular serine proteases of *Dermatophilus congolensis* isolates from cattle, sheep and horses. *Veterinary Microbiology* 62, 321–335.

Weese, J.S. and Yu, A.A. (2013) Infectious folliculitis and dermatophytosis. *Veterinary Clinics of North America: Equine Practice* 29, 559–575.

Pemphigus foliaceus

Leclere, M. (2017) Corticosteroids and immune suppressive therapies in horses. *Veterinary Clinics of North America: Equine Practice* 33, 17–27.

Rosenkrantz, W. (2013) Immune-mediated dermatoses. *Veterinary Clinics of North America: Equine Practice* 29, 607–613.

Vandenabeele, S.I., White, S.D., Affolter, V.K., Kass, P.H. and Ihrke, P.J. (2004) Pemphigus foliaceus in the horse: a retrospective study of 20 cases. *Veterinary Dermatology* 15, 381–388.

White, S.D., Maxwell, L.K., Szabo, N.J., Hawkins, J.L. and Kollias-Baker, C. (2005) Pharmacokinetics of azathioprine following single-dose intravenous and oral administration and effects of azathioprine following chronic oral administration in horses. *American Journal of Veterinary Research* 66, 1578–1583.

White, S.D., Rosychuk, R.A., Outerbridge, C.A., Fieseler, K.V., Spier, S. *et al.* (2000) Thiopurine methyltransferase in red blood cells of dogs, cats, and horses. *Journal of Veterinary Internal Medicine* 14, 499–502.

Zabel, S., Mueller, R.S., Fieseler, K.V., Bettenay, S.V., Littlewood, J.D. and Wagner, R. (2005) Review of 15 cases of pemphigus foliaceus in horses and a survey of the literature. *Veterinary Record* 157, 505–509.

Equine sarcoidosis

Sloet van Oldruitenborgh-Oosterbaan, M.M. and Grinwis, G.C. (2013) Equine sarcoidosis. *Veterinary Clinics of North America: Equine Practice* 29, 615–627.

Sloet van Oldruitenborgh-Oosterbaan, M.M. and Grinwis, G.C. (2013) Equine sarcoidosis: clinical signs, diagnosis, treatment and outcome of 22 cases. *Veterinary Dermatology* 24, 218–224.e48.

8 Clinical Approach to Nodular Diseases

Many diseases present with nodular dermatitis in horses ranging from allergic to infectious, and thus it is important to have a systematic approach to achieve the correct diagnosis and recommend the appropriate treatment. Some of the most common differential diagnoses are listed in Table 8.1. Some are sterile diseases, while others are infectious or neoplastic. It is important to consider the age of the patient, the distribution of the lesions, and the progression and presence of systemic clinical signs in order to rank the differential diagnoses.

In the initial evaluation, cytology should be done on any draining lesion, with the knowledge that the organisms observed on the surface may not be representative of the deeper pathological process and that this test may not be diagnostic in some cases. Biopsy should be considered in most cases. If possible, the biopsy should be done by taking intact nodules that have not yet ruptured as these may be more representative of the underlying process. The sample should be split and submitted for both histopathology and culture if an infectious disease is suspected (Fig. 8.1). In this chapter, the focus will be on non-neoplastic differential diagnoses for nodular dermatitis in horses and the diagnostic approach for this type of clinical presentation.

Infectious Causes of Nodules

Fungal diseases

Fungal diseases may be primarily cutaneous when the infection occurs due to inoculation of the fungus in the skin or systemic when the cutaneous nodules represent the spreading to the skin of a systemic disease. Subcutaneous infections are acquired by contamination of a wound with the fungal organism. Many of these are saprophytic fungi present in soil. Systemic fungal infections are typically acquired by inhalation and the patient will show systemic signs of illness.

Sporotrichosis

Sporothrix schenckii is a dimorphic saprophyte found in the environment, in the soil and on plants such as thorny bushes. It occurs worldwide and is a common saprophyte of decaying plant material. Infection results from inoculation of the organism into the subcutaneous tissue via accidental pricking with thorns where the organism is present. In its saprophytic stage or when cultured at 25°C, *Sporothrix* is present in the filamentous stage, which is composed of hyphae and conidia, while in tissue it is visible as the yeast form. The yeast-like cells may be various sizes and shapes. They may be round to oval, with a diameter of 2–6 μm, and usually have elongated, cigar-shaped buds on a narrow base.

Sporotrichosis is uncommon and is more likely to occur in tropical climates. It is an example of a fungal cutaneous nodular disease, as the infection is usually acquired through the skin and primarily affects the skin and lymphatics, only rarely spreading to internal organs.

This disease is zoonotic, and infection can occur in people by contamination of an open wound with the exudate of an infected animal. Nodules appear first at the site of inoculation. Over time, the fungus spreads through the lymph vessels causing palpable thickening or "cording" of the lymphatic chain surrounding the primary lesion. Regional lymph nodes can become involved. The nodules eventually become large, ulcerate and drain serosanguinous fluid. Lesions are found most commonly on the extremities, and multiple nodules may be present along the lymphatic vessel (Fig. 8.2). Sometimes, lesions are present on the neck. The nodules are non-pruritic, firm, non-painful and can release a purulent exudate when they ulcerate. The disease sometimes has a waxing and waning course with periods of new lesions developing intermingled with periods of improvement. Sporotrichosis should be suspected in any case of lymphangitis. Other differential diagnoses

Table 8.1. Common differential diagnoses of nodular diseases in horses.

Infectious diseases		Sterile inflammatory diseases	Neoplastic diseases
Infectious agent	Example		
Fungal		Eosinophilic granuloma	Sarcoids
Subcutaneous	Sporotrichosis	Foreign body	Melanoma
	Opportunistic infection, e.g. phaeohyphomycosis	Sarcoidosis	Mast cell tumor
Systemic	Cryptococcosis	Nodular panniculitis	Basal cell tumor
Oomyces	*Pythium*		Lymphoma
Parasitic	*Habronema*		Glandular tumors
Bacterial	*Mycobacterium* (e.g. atypical mycobacteria)		Cysts
	Staphylococcus (e.g. furunculosis)		Other tumors
	Nocardia		
	Actinomyces		
	Actinobacillus		
Protozoal	*Leishmania*		

Diagnostic approach to nodular diseases in horses

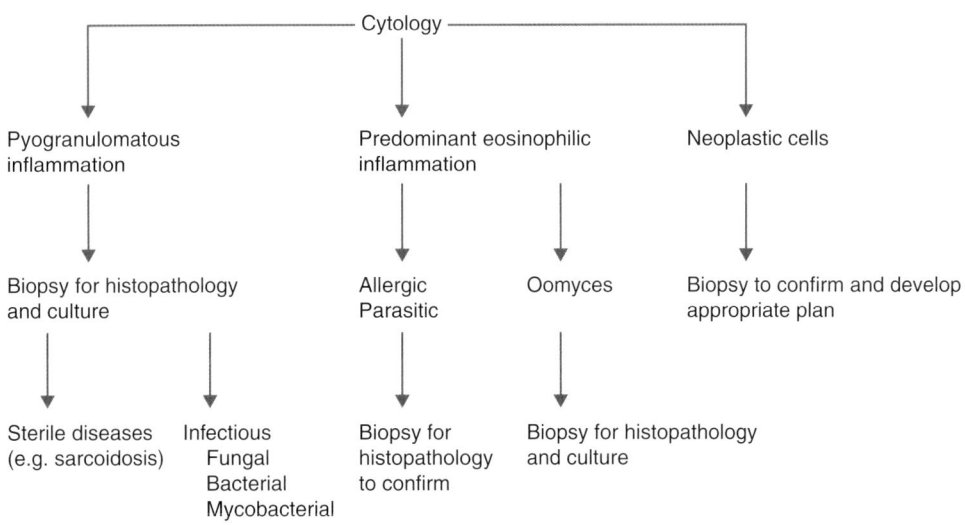

Fig. 8.1. The diagnostic approach to nodular dermatitis in horses. It is important to discriminate between infections and sterile diseases. Sterile diseases may be either inflammatory or neoplastic.

should be bacterial infections such as glanders (caused by *Pseudomonas mallei*), ulcerative lymphangitic (caused by *Corynebacterium pseudotuberculosis*) and systemic fungal infections (e.g. *Histoplasma farciminosum*).

The organisms may be seen on cytology together with a pyogranulomatous exudate. In horses, the organisms typically are not abundant, so it is possible to miss them on cytology. It is important to emphasize that whenever a pyogranulomatous exudate is present, an infectious cause should be considered, and that failure to detect organisms does not rule out the possibility of infection. This is why the history and clinical presentation are crucial in orienting the clinician toward the primary differential diagnosis.

Biopsy of an intact nodule and histopathology using special stains (e.g. Gridley or Giemsa) may help in increasing the chances of a diagnosis. The organism may be difficult to find in tissues, even

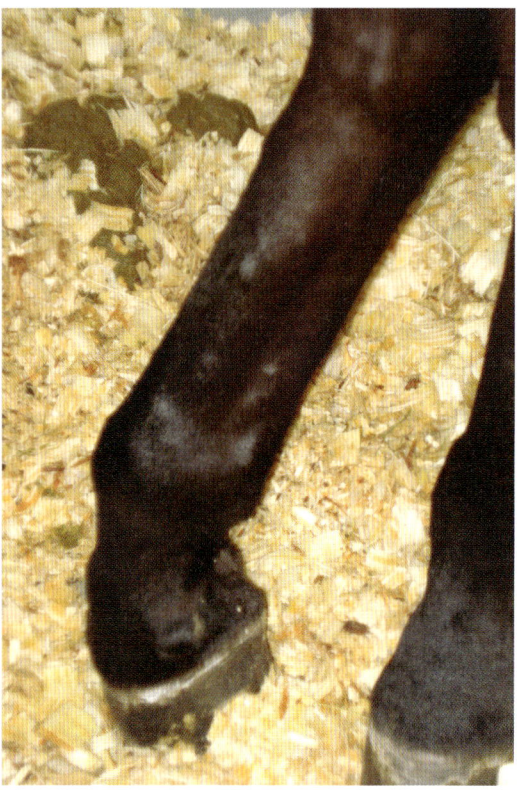

Fig. 8.2. Sporotrichosis on the leg of a horse. The nodules have developed progressively over time following a linear course

with special stains making this diagnosis challenging. PCR has been used to diagnose sporotrichosis in other species. Biopsy samples can also be cultured on Sabouraud agar. Serum antibodies can also be investigated.

Treatment of affected horses typically involves the use of 20% sodium iodide, given at 20–40 mg/kg/day intravenously (IV) for 2–5 days, and then at 1–2 mg/kg PO twice daily for 1 week, followed by 0.5–1.0 mg/kg PO once daily. Treatment should be continued for 30 days beyond clinical cure. Another option is potassium iodide (10 mg/kg PO once daily). Typically, a minimum of 1 month is necessary to see regression of the lesions. Adverse effects are known as iodism and include scaling, alopecia, dull mentation, anorexia, fever, coughing, lacrimation, serous nasal discharge, salivation, nervousness and cardiovascular abnormalities. If iodism is observed, the drug should be stopped for 1 week and then reinstituted at a lower dose.

Deep mycoses (blastomycosis, coccidioidomycosis, cryptococcosis, histoplasmosis)

Deep mycoses are fungal infections of internal organs that disseminate hematogenously to the skin. The animal inhales the conidia, which then spread via the blood. Primary inoculation into the skin is rare. Demonstrating the organism by cytology of direct smears or tissue aspirates, or by histopathology (by using special stains), is sufficient to make a diagnosis for all deep mycoses. Attempts at culture should be done with care due to the risk of transmission to laboratory technicians. Serology has been used to confirm the diagnosis and to increase the likelihood of diagnosis in the event that negative results are found on cytology or biopsy.

Blastomycosis is caused by *Blastomyces dermatitidis*, a dimorphic saprophytic fungus. This disease is reported primarily in North America in specific areas (Illinois, Mississippi, Missouri, New York and Ohio). Therefore, when considering horses, it is important to inquire about travel history.

Coccidioides immitis, the cause of coccidioidomycosis, is also a dimorphic saprophytic fungus. In the USA, this organism is typical of sandy, dry areas such as Mexico and some parts of the south-western USA. Infection is rare in horses, but travel to an endemic area should raise suspicion of this differential diagnosis. Infection occurs by inhalation and rarely by direct inoculation of the organism into the skin. Again, culturing should be limited to appropriately equipped laboratories. Serology tests are commonly used to make a diagnosis, and immunodiffusion, enzyme immunoassays or antigen-coated latex particle agglutination have been used for *Coccidioides*. Serial testing can give a sense of the prognosis, as falling titers indicate improvement while increasing titers indicate worsening of the disease. Fluconazole is considered the drug of choice for coccidiomycosis with a loading dose of 14 mg/kg PO, followed by 5 mg/kg PO once daily. The correct duration of treatment is important and can vary from patient to patient. Care should be used when handling the exudate of affected horses as cross-infection has been reported. Bleach kills the arthroconidia of this fungus and should be used to decontaminate infected material.

Cryptococcosis is caused by a ubiquitous, saprophytic, yeast-like fungus and has been reported in all continents. Fungi of the *Cryptococcus gattii/ Cryptococcus neoformans* species complex can cause respiratory disease in horses. *C. neoformans* var. *neoformans* is more prevalent in the USA and Europe, while *C. neoformans* var. *gattii* is more common in Australia, Africa and South America. Infection occurs by inhalation and rarely by direct inoculation of the organism into the skin. Affected horses in the majority of cases are otherwise immunocompetent. *C gattii* occurs with greater frequency than *C. neoformans* in equine pulmonary cryptococcosis and can be treated successfully with enteral fluconazole monotherapy, with disease severity determining treatment length. For cryptococcosis, both lateral flow assays and later cryptococcal antigen titer are used for diagnosis and monitoring of treatment. The lateral flow assay has the advantage that it can be performed quickly with minimal training and uses antibodies to detect the cryptococcal capsule antigens of all species of *Cryptococcus* and thus is very sensitive for all serotypes. Fluconazole has been used successfully as monotherapy for cryptococcosis in horses. Due to the oral administration and the reasonable cost compared with other treatment options, it is a good alternative to consider.

Histoplasmosis (epizootic lymphangitis) is caused by the dimorphic fungus *Histoplasma capsulatum* var. *farciminosum*. This disease is endemic in Africa, and Asia. Horses and mules are the major reservoir for this infection (up to 39% have been reported to be infected in Ethiopia), which is facilitated by trauma from biting insects. The organism can survive for up to 10 weeks in the environment, so infected bedding can act as a source of infection. The disease manifests as a nodular eruption. Various forms are described, and the disease can range from asymptomatic to ocular, cutaneous and respiratory. The nodules are initially firm but over time can become softer and rupture, releasing an infected purulent exudate. The nodules may follow the lymphatics and eventually tend to spread toward the inguinal area. Horses are initially systemically unaffected, but with chronicity, this disease can lead to weight loss and poor overall health. Diagnosis is made by cytological examination of the exudate, which reveals the organisms inside macrophages. A more sensitive and specific test is the use of PCR on blood and aspirates of the nodules. Sodium iodide and potassium iodide are most commonly used for treatment of this disease.

Oomycotic infections

The most common oomycetes that cause infections are *Pythium insidiosum* and *Lagenidium* spp. These are not true fungi because they lack ergosterol in their cell wall. Oomycetes also lack chitin in the cell wall. They are plant parasites and can be found in standing water that contains decaying plant material. They cause infection after the zoospores invade traumatized skin. Infections are more commonly reported in the tropics and subtropics. In the USA, this infection is common in the southern states, frequently in late summer and fall after heavy rains. Minor microtrauma has been shown to be sufficient to allow penetration. The infective stage of *P. insidiosum* is a zoospore, which is motile and has an affinity for animal hair and cut edges of the skin. Infection can develop from standing in or drinking infected water. Infected animals are otherwise immunocompetent and healthy, so no immune suppression is necessary to contract this disease. The immune response built toward the oomycetes, however, is critical in determining whether an infection will occur after exposure or not. It is currently believed that a humoral response leads to infection while a cell-mediated response is critical for resolution or resistance toward the development of the infection.

Ulcerated nodules can be seen on the face (Fig. 8.3), distal limbs (Figs 8.4 and 8.5), thorax and ventral abdomen. Occasionally, nodules occur elsewhere on the body. The nodules swell and then drain a thick, stringy exudate. The lesions are deep and often involve the subcutis. They are usually very pruritic and rapidly increase in size. This may be why this disease used to be referred to as "swamp cancer."

Kunkers are often found within the nodule and are exuded together with the exudate. Kunkers are hard masses containing *Pythium* hyphae surrounded by profound eosinophilic inflammation, necrotic tissue and blood vessels. Kunkers most likely represent the immune system's attempt to wall off the organism and extrude it from the lesion. Over time, *Pythium* will invade underlying structures such as vessels, bones, the trachea and the lungs. It may also spread through the lymphatics to distant sites. A gastrointestinal form has also been described, manifesting as colic and the presence of intestinal granulomas.

Cytology and biopsy of the nodules are helpful to make a tentative diagnosis. Histopathology shows a massive eosinophilic infiltrate (Fig. 8.6) in which clear spaces shaped like hyphae ("ghost figures") are visible (Fig. 8.7). Special stains (e.g. GMS) help to visualize wide, sparsely septate hyphae (Fig. 8.8) consistent with oomycetes, and this supports the

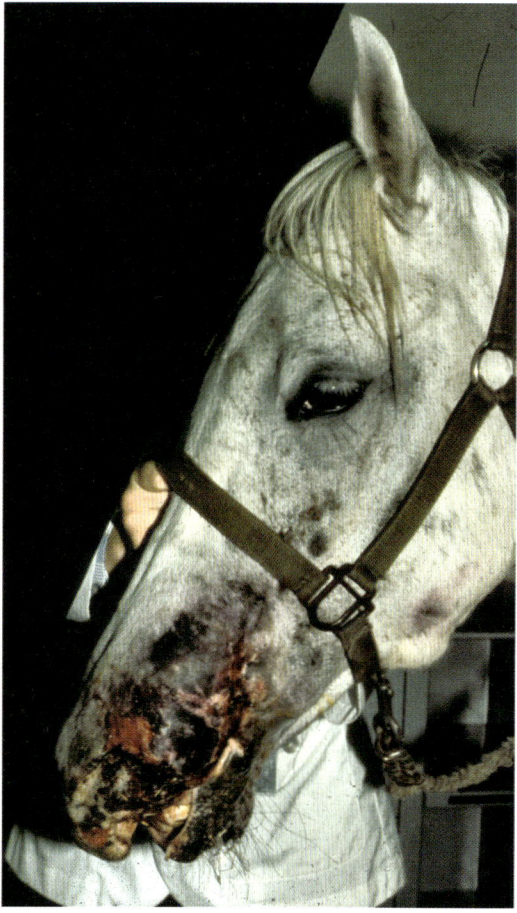

Fig. 8.3. *Pythium* infection on the face of a horse. Infection in this case occurred by exposure to contaminated drinking water. (Courtesy of Large Animal Service, University of Florida.)

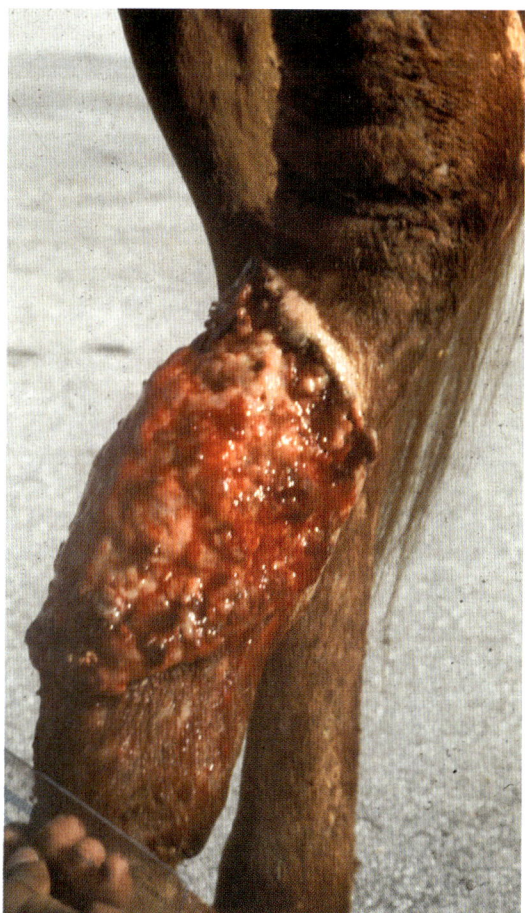

Fig. 8.4. Severe pythiosis on the leg of a horse. In this case, the infection had progressed from cutaneous to involvement of the bone. This horse was euthanized due to the extent and severity of its disease.

diagnosis. Detection on histopathology, however, is not sufficient to make a final diagnosis, as it does not allow differentiation from other organisms such as zygomycetes (causing zygomycosis). The final diagnosis is made by culture of the tissue or, preferably, of the kunkers. It is important to handle the samples properly to increase the likelihood of a positive culture. Samples should be unrefrigerated, if possible, and shipped to the laboratory to be used for culture in less than 24 h. Serology has also been used for the diagnosis of pythiosis. This type of approach is not 100% specific, and false-positive results may be seen for other fungal infections. PCR from tissues can also be done to obtain a specific diagnosis, as well as immunohistochemistry using polyclonal antibodies for *Pythium* in tissue.

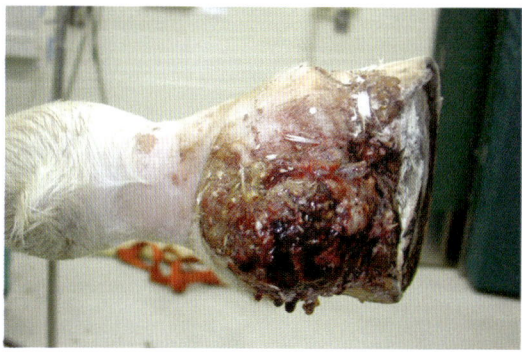

Fig. 8.5. Large *Pythium* lesion on the pastern of a horse that had spent time in a flooded paddock after a hurricane.

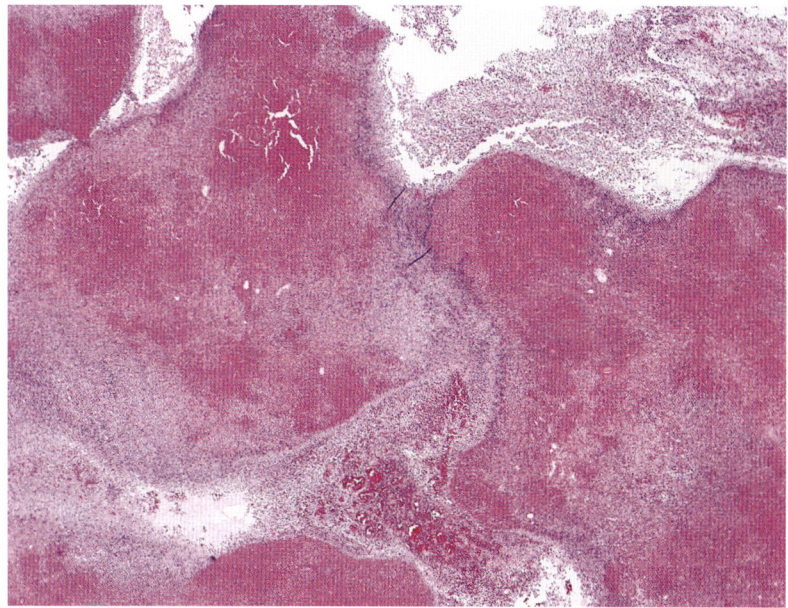

Fig. 8.6. Histopathology of a *Pythium* case. Note the severe inflammatory response completely obliterating the normal structure of the skin (100× magnification). (Courtesy of Dr William Craft, University of Florida.)

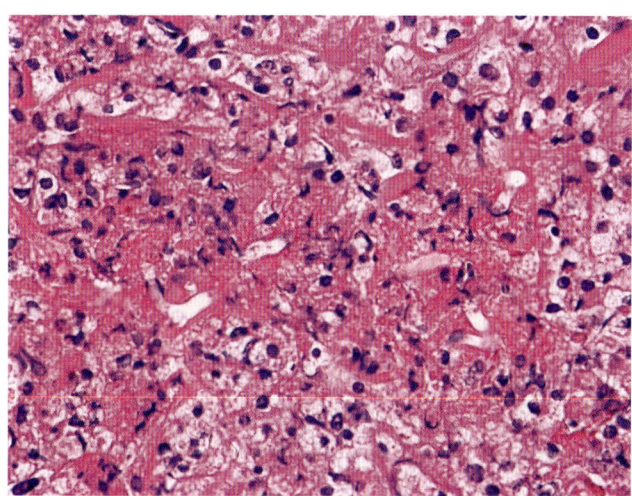

Fig. 8.7. "Ghost figures" (clear spaces in the shape of hyphae) can be seen in the inflammatory infiltrate of this case of pythiosis (1000× magnification). (Courtesy of Dr William Craft, University of Florida.)

Early diagnosis is critical for treatment success. The prognosis is guarded if detected early and grave if detected late (more than 3 months). Immunotherapy has been used to modulate the immune response and encourage a cell-mediated response. Several formulations have been developed over the years. It is important to note that, although the term "vaccine" is frequently used for these preparations, they are not used for prevention; instead, they are used for treatment in horses that have already developed the infection. These preparations are more effective the earlier the diagnosis, with cure rates close to 100% if the infection has been present for less than 2 weeks. Failure is typically seen in cases that have had the infection for more than 2 months. The most currently used vaccine contains both secreted antigens and soluble mycelial antigens. The protocol consists of multiple injections (an initial intradermal

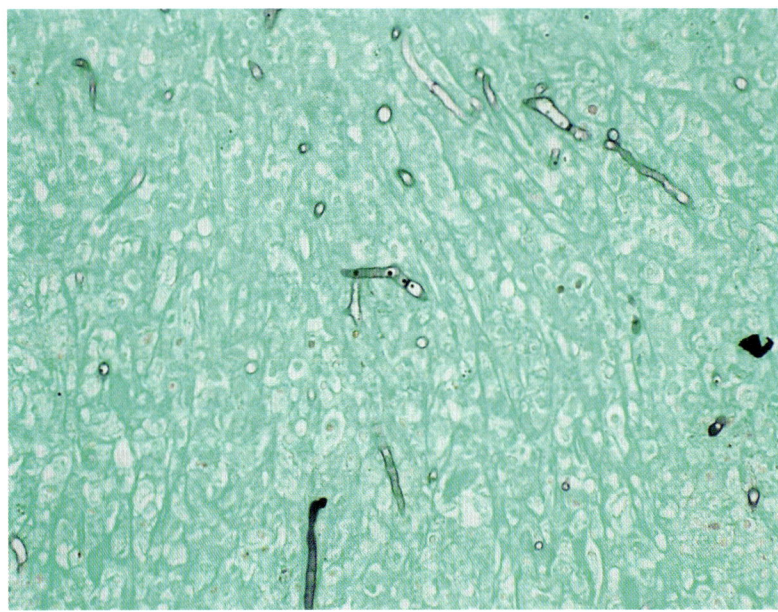

Fig. 8.8. A special stain (GMS) allows visualization of hyphae consistent with pythiosis (600× magnification). (Courtesy of Dr William Craft, University of Florida.)

injection of 0.1 ml, followed by a subcutaneous injection after 2 weeks). If necessary, additional injections can be given weekly for up to 2 months. Horses that develop large reactions at the site of the injections are typically those that will respond favorably to the immunotherapy. The vaccine is much more likely to achieve success if the lesions are less than 2 weeks old and if combined with surgical debulking. It can be purchased from Pan American Veterinary Laboratories (http://pythium.pavlab.com/).

Surgery is recommended as the best option for treatment, wherever possible. Ideally, 2–3 cm margins are preferred to avoid recurrence. Unfortunately, these margins are often not possible and surgical resection is incomplete, requiring additional treatments such as immunotherapy or use of a hyperbaric chamber.

Medical therapy is typically ineffective, as *Pythium* lacks ergosterol, which is the target of antifungal drugs such as azoles, terbinafine and amphotericin B. Photodynamic therapy and a hyperbaric chamber can be considered as adjunctive options for pythiosis and anecdotally have been reported to yield a very good response.

Eumycotic mycetoma

Eumycotic mycetomas are caused by soil saprophytes, which are inoculated into the dermis by wound contamination. The most common fungi isolated are *Pseudallescheria boydii* (which produces white granules) and *Curvularia geniculata* (which produces black granules). Horses present with large, swollen nodules and draining tracts with granules in the discharge. The lesions are usually solitary and are found most commonly on the distal limbs and face. Differential diagnoses include foreign body granulomas, other infectious causes and neoplasia. Diagnosis is made by first performing cytology of the exudate, as hyphae are easily seen by crushing the granules and staining the slide. Skin biopsies for histopathology and fungal culture are recommended for definitive diagnosis. The treatment of choice is wide-margin surgical excision, which is typically curative. If complete margins are not achieved, itraconazole 3 mg/kg PO twice daily may be attempted and should be continued for 2–3 months after clinical cure.

Phaeohyphomycosis

Phaeohyphomycosis is caused by a group of ubiquitous saprophytic fungi that are inoculated through a wound. These fungi form pigmented hyphal elements but do not form granules (in contrast to eumycotic mycetomas). Many fungi have been isolated in this disease but the most common organisms are *Alternaria alternaria*, *Bipolaris specifera* and *Cladosporium* spp. The lesions are typically firm, well-circumscribed dermal nodules that tend to spread progressively from the area of inoculation (Fig. 8.9). Diagnosis is made by cytology, histopathology and fungal culture. The treatment of choice is wide-margin surgical excision. Spontaneous remission has been reported after 3 months. The response to systemic antifungal therapy is unpredictable and depends on the specific fungus responsible for the infection. Therefore, it is important to biopsy and culture these lesions and to request an antifungal sensitivity panel from the laboratory.

Zygomycosis

Zygomycetes are ubiquitous soil saprophytes and can be found as a normal part of the flora of the skin and hair coat in horses. The portal of entry when they cause disease may be gastrointestinal, respiratory or by wound contamination. This

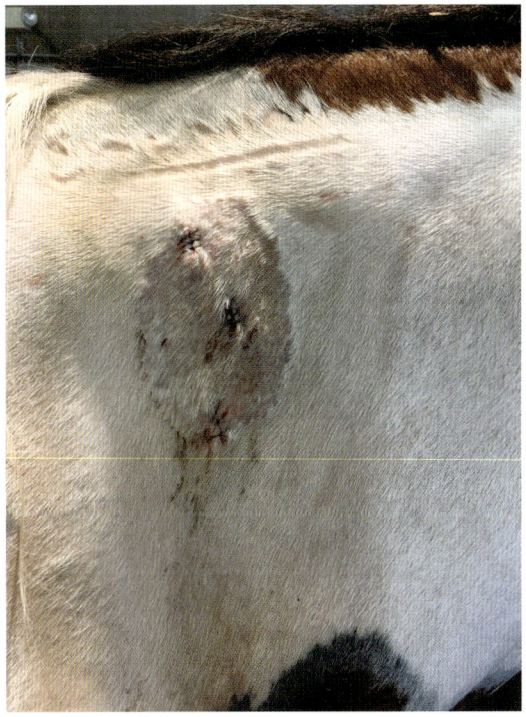

Fig. 8.9. Phaeohyphomycosis on the lateral neck of a horse, believed to have started with an injection. The lesions had spread over the course of several months. Alopecia has spread centrifugally, and several nodules have developed to involve an increasingly larger area.

disease is more common in the tropics and subtropics. The two orders of zygmoycetes that cause disease are: (i) *Mucorales*, including *Rhizopus* and *Mucor* spp.; and (ii) *Entomophthorales*, including *Conidiobolus* and *Basidiobolus* spp. The clinical signs are large, annular, ulcerated nodules that drain serosanguinous fluid. They may be single or multiple. *Conidiobolus* lesions are found most commonly on the external nares and nasal passages. *Basidiobolus* lesions are more commonly found on the thorax, trunk, head and neck. Diagnosis is confirmed by cytology, histopathology and fungal culture. Treatment includes wide-margin surgical excision, followed by amphotericin B or potassium iodide.

Bacterial diseases

Staphylococcus

Staphylococcus infection is usually associated with a solitary abscess in a site of previous trauma or surgery. It is prudent always to wear gloves and to perform cytology of the exudate. If cocci are seen on cytology, a swab of the purulent exudate should be taken and submitted for aerobic culture. This is important because MRSA is a problem in horses and may cause disease in people. Resistance has been increasingly reported in the field (see Chapter 7 on bacterial folliculitis) and therefore clinicians need to be mindful about proper antibiotic use and the potential for transmission of this pattern of resistance to people.

Horses with MRSA need to be isolated from all other horses, and people who have contact with them must wear full protective clothing – gloves, a gown and a mask. MRSA requires systemic antibiotic therapy based on culture results, lancing of the abscess and flushing with sterile saline/povidone or saline/chlorhexidine solution. The horse should be isolated and a contact prevention protocol followed until clinical signs have resolved and the horse has at least one negative culture. People who touched or handled the horse should be evaluated by their physician for MRSA carriage.

Streptococcus

Streptococcus can cause several diseases in horses. It is reported to cause ulcerative lymphangitis and folliculitis, and is the cause of strangles, a disease of the upper respiratory tract in horses; it also causes abscess in the mandibular area and local lymph nodes. A hypersensitivity reaction to *Streptococcus* is also associated with purpura hemorrhagica. Therefore, this organism is of great importance in equine medicine. Cytology should always be done when lancing equine abscesses. Swabs should also be taken and submitted for culture and sensitivity. The majority of *Streptococcus* strains are sensitive to penicillin and oral sulfonamides.

Corynebacterium

Corynebacterium can cause nodular diseases in horses. In particular, *C. pseudotuberculosis* is the cause of pigeon breast, also known as Wyoming strangles. The organism is transmitted by biting flies and typically causes large, single abscesses on the lateral thorax or chest of horses (Figs 8.10 and 8.11). When the abscess matures and drains, the exudate is caseous and yellow (Fig. 8.12). It is mostly diagnosed in the warmer months and the incubation time is 2–4 weeks. After drainage, the lesions heal slowly, leaving ulcerated or scarred areas (Figs 8.13 and 8.14). Drainage and systemic antibiotics are necessary to cure the lesions. The organism is typically sensitive to penicillin and oral sulfonamides.

Occasionally, *C. pseudotuberculosis* infection can progress causing lymphangitis. Luckily, with improved management and hygiene, these cases are now extremely rare. Other organisms that can cause ulcerative lymphangitis are *Pseudomonas*, *Histoplasma*, *Pasteurella* and *Actinomyces* spp. Cytology and culture of the exudate are important

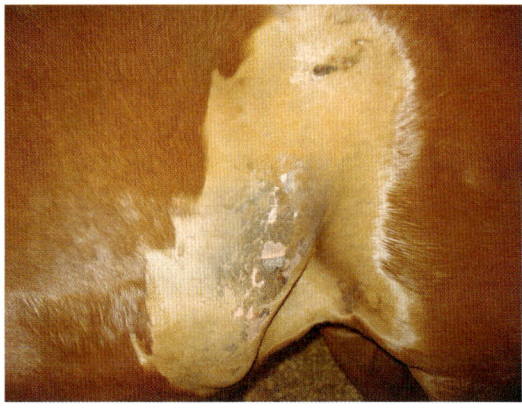

Fig. 8.10. *Corynebacterium pseudotuberculosis* infection on the side of a horse. The large nodules/ abscess had developed quickly and required draining ventrally.

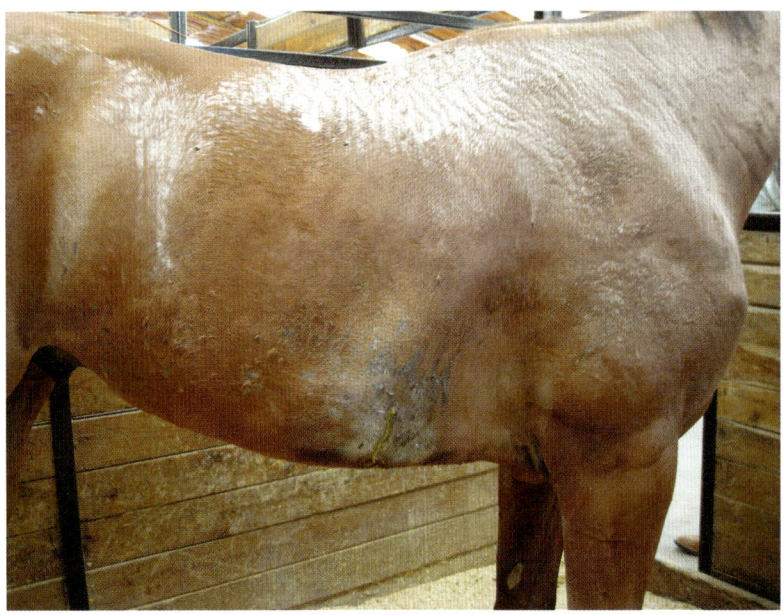

Fig. 8.11. Another case of *Corynebacterium pseudotuberculosis* infection where the abscess is starting to drain yellow, purulent material.

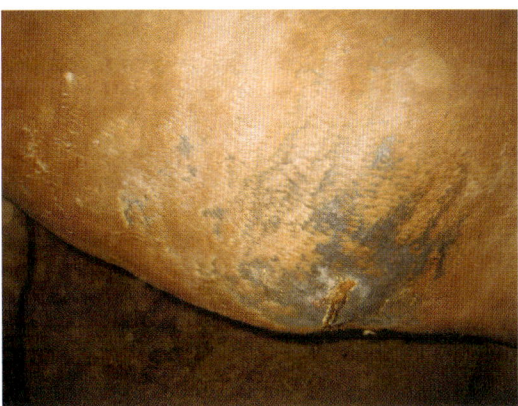

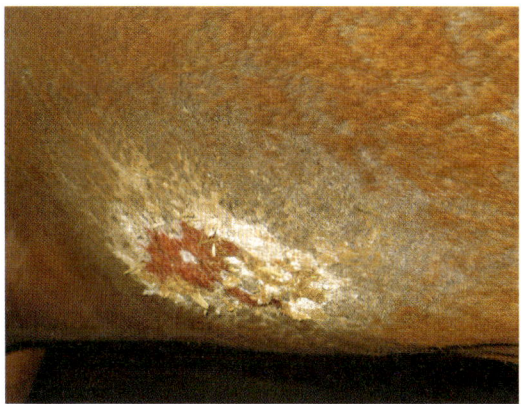

Fig. 8.12. Close-up of the abscess of the horse shown in Fig. 8.11.

Fig. 8.13. Close-up of the horse shown in Fig. 8.11, showing the progression to ulcerative lesions.

for proper identification of the cause and the most appropriate treatment.

Glanders

This is a largely fatal bacterial disease of horses in Africa and Asia. It is caused by *Burkholderia mallei*. This bacterium was previously classified as a *Pseudomonas* sp. This is a Gram-negative, obligate aerobic, rod-shaped bacterium that establishes infection following ingestion of contaminated feed or water. The acute phase is typically fatal in a few days. Horses show signs of respiratory disease, cough and fever and the release of an infectious nasal discharge, followed by septicemia and death within days. Horses that survive become carriers. For this reason, this is a **reportable disease** in most of the world and treatment is often forbidden. In the chronic form, nasal and subcutaneous nodules develop, eventually ulcerating.

Parasitic diseases

Cutaneous habronemiasis (summer sores)

Horses are parasitized by three nematode species: *Habronema muscae*, *Habronema majus* and *Draschia megastoma*. The adults reside in the stomach where they cause little reaction; the exception is *D. megastoma*, which produces varying-sized nodules that usually occur near the margo plicatus. When the larvae penetrate damaged skin, they incite a hypersensitivity reaction, resulting in cutaneous habronemiasis. This disease sometimes develops in horses with wounds; once they get it, recurrence is common year after year unless stringent preventative measures are taken. The disease is seasonal, first appearing in the spring, and most cases clear spontaneously in the winter. Disease occurrence is sporadic, and only a few horses in any given area will be affected.

The lesions usually involve the medial canthus of the eye, the male genitalia (especially the urethral process) and the lower extremities (wounds) (see Chapter 6, this volume). The lesions comprise areas of granulation tissue containing small, gritty, yellow nodules (Figs 8.15–8.18). These lesions are very large in donkeys and mules. Differential diagnoses for this type of presentation include exuberant granulation tissue (proud flesh), fibroblastic sarcoid, squamous cell carcinoma, pythiosis (phycomycosis) and zygomycosis.

Diagnosis is made by histopathology and detection of the parasite in the dermis (see Chapter 6, this volume). The aim of treatment is to reduce the size of the lesions, decrease inflammation and prevent reinfection. The larvae will die anyway (larval death may be part of pathogenesis), so killing them may not be important. Due to the recurrent nature of the disease, strict attention should be paid to fly control and immediate wound care in future years to decrease the chances of reinfection. Affected horses are allergic to the parasites, so subsequent exposure to the larvae will trigger a more severe inflammatory response.

Treatment is systemic ivermectin combined with surgical debulking and intralesional or systemically administered corticosteroids to reduce the inflammation. Intralesional triamcinolone (5–15 mg/lesion) can

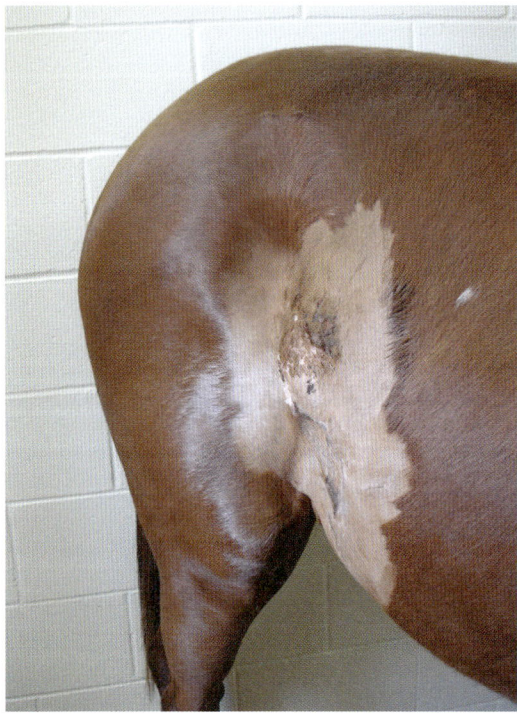

Fig. 8.14. The same horse as that shown in Fig. 8.11 after the lesions had been drained. Note the large area of scarring.

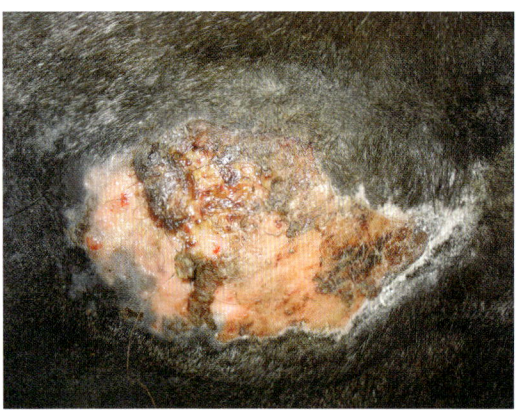

Fig. 8.15. *Habronema* infection on the side of a horse. The lesion had grown slowly and was very pruritic.

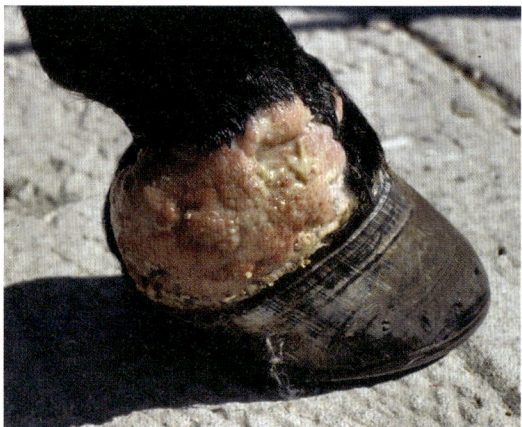

Fig. 8.16. *Habronema* infection on the pastern. This horse had a history of "recurrent summer sores."

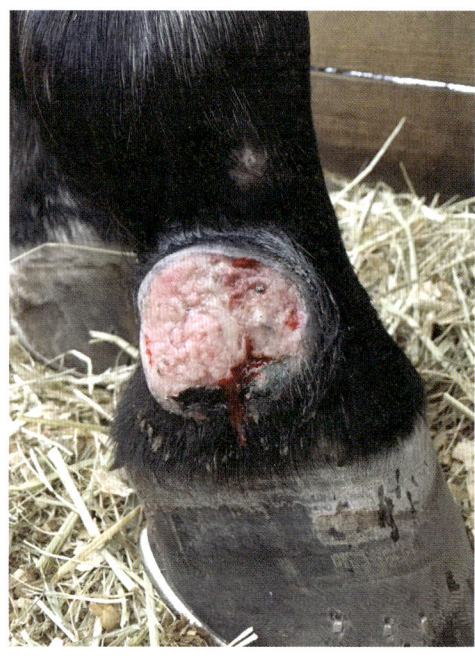

Fig. 8.17. Severe habronemiasis in which surgical debridement had been attempted but lesions kept recurring.

be used without exceeding a total body dose of 20 mg. If several lesions are present, systemic prednisolone 400 mg/day for 10–14 days can be prescribed to decrease pruritus and the inflammatory response against the parasite.

Sterile Inflammatory Causes of Nodules

Eosinophilic granuloma

This disease is also called equine collagenolytic granuloma with collagen degeneration. There is no apparent breed, age or sex predilection. The most prominent feature of the disease is degeneration of collagen; however, the pathogenesis probably involves a hypersensitivity reaction. Both nematode larvae and insect bites have been suggested as possible causes, but there is no real evidence to substantiate this. The disease usually occurs during the warmer months of the year, but some stables report it in winter. The lesions consist of one to several firm nodules situated in the dermis (Fig. 8.19).

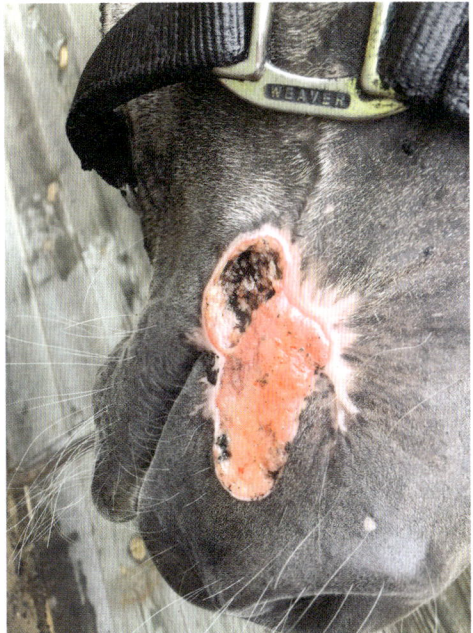

Fig. 8.18. The healing stages of habronemiasis in a patient that had undergone surgical resection and has developed scarring.

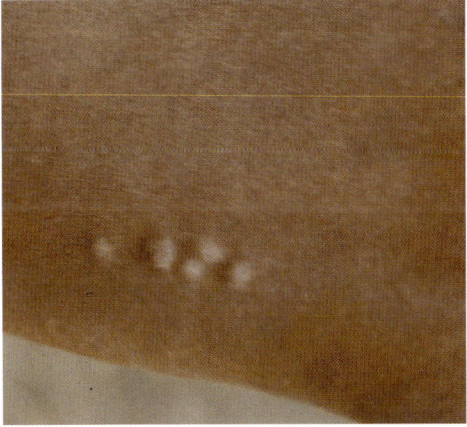

Fig. 8.19. Eosinophilic granulomas in an insect-allergic horse. The nodules are hard and non-pruritic.

A generalized form on the face, neck and thorax occurs in Arab horses.

The nodules vary from 0.5 to 5 cm in diameter. The overlying skin surface and hair coat are normal in appearance. The nodules usually occur on the sides of the neck, the withers and the back. There is no pruritus associated with this disease. Diagnosis is made by biopsy (total excision) of a lesion for histopathology.

Treatment consists of prednisolone 1–2 mg/kg PO daily for 2–3 weeks; the dose is then slowly decreased. Mineralized lesions will not disappear completely with steroid therapy. In some horses, additional lesions may subsequently develop after the corticosteroid therapy is discontinued, necessitating retreatment. There is some indication that the lesions may regress spontaneously with time. If there are only a few lesions, sublesional triamcinolone acetonide is probably the treatment of choice; use 5 mg per lesion (maximum total dose of 20 mg) two to three times at 10-day intervals. Surgical excision is curative for solitary lesions.

Other Nodular Diseases

Many neoplastic diseases can affect the skin. An in-depth discussion of neoplastic diseases is beyond the scope of this chapter. Diagnosis of these diseases requires a biopsy for histopathology. One special consideration is for sarcoids. This is one of the most common and locally aggressive forms of cutaneous tumor. Many presentations occur, ranging from benign to aggressive and ulcerative presentations. It is important to emphasize that the occult form of sarcoid (Fig. 8.20) should not be biopsied or traumatized to avoid progression into more aggressive forms. Some presentations of sarcoids are shown in Figs 8.21 and 8.22. It is believed that flies may play a role in the transmission of papillomavirus, which has been implicated in the pathogenesis of some forms of sarcoids. The ears appear to be a commonly affected area (Fig. 8.23).

All other types of cutaneous tumor should be biopsied to be properly diagnosed and to formulate an appropriate treatment plan and establish an accurate prognosis.

Conclusions and Take Home Messages

Nodular dermatitis is common in horses and can be triggered by a variety of conditions ranging from infectious to sterile. Depending on the age, travel history, appearance and progression of disease, various

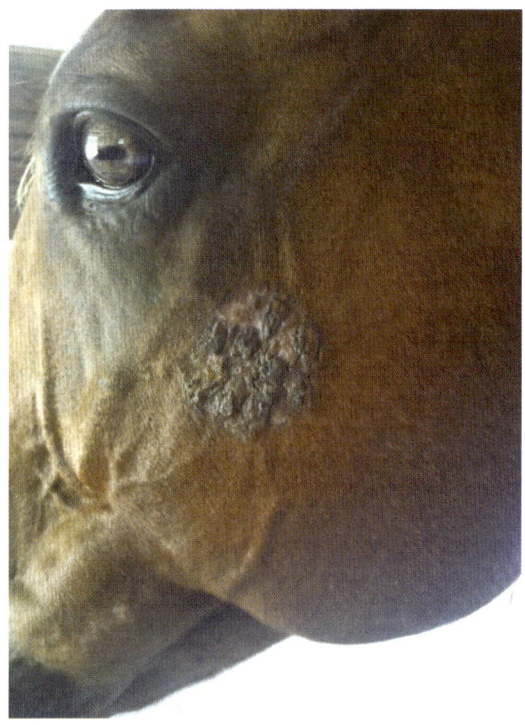

Fig. 8.20. An occult sarcoid on the face of a horse.

differential diagnoses should be considered. It is crucial to rule out infectious diseases, especially in warm climates where infections are more common. Cytology of the exudate and a biopsy for histopathology, culture and sensitivity is indicated in most cases.

Further Reading

Sporotrichosis

Crothers, S.L., White, S.D., Ihrke, P.J. and Affolter, V.K. (2009) Sporotrichosis: a retrospective evaluation of 23 cases seen in northern California (1987–2007). *Veterinary Dermatology* 20, 249–259.

de Lima Barros, M.B., de Almeida Paes, R. and Schubach, A.O. (2011) *Sporothrix schenckii* and sporotrichosis. *Clinical Microbiology Reviews* 24, 633–654.

White, S.D. (2005) Equine bacterial and fungal diseases: a diagnostic and therapeutic update. *Clinical Techniques in Equine Practice* 4, 302–310.

Systemic fungal infections

Kinne, J., Joseph, M., Wernery, U., Nogradi, N. and Hagen, F. (2017) Disseminated *Cryptococcus deuterogattii* (AFLP6/VGII) infection in an Arabian horse

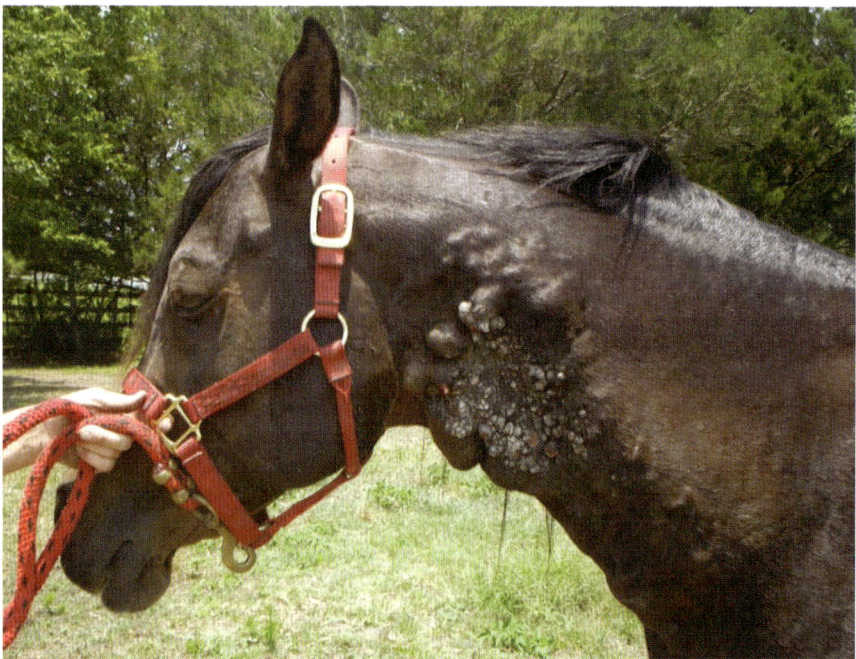

Fig. 8.21. A mixed verrucous and fibroblastic sarcoid.

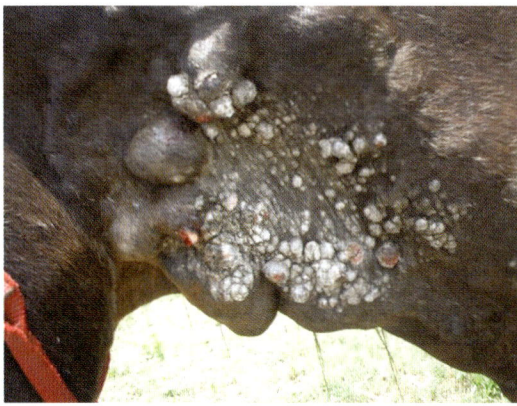

Fig. 8.22. Close-up of the lesions on the patient shown in Fig. 8.21.

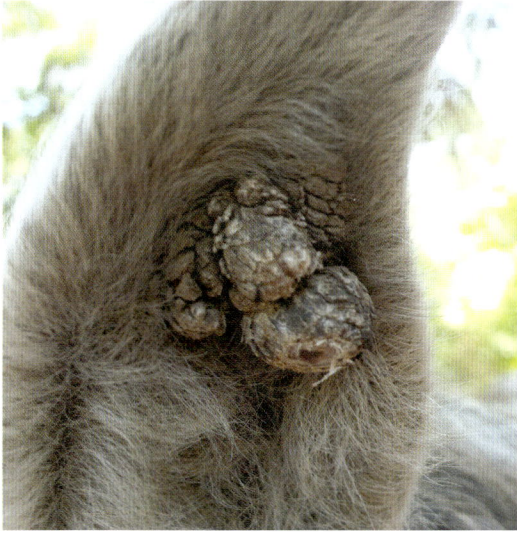

Fig. 8.23. A verrucous sarcoid on the pinna.

from Dubai, United Arab Emirates. *Revista Iberoamericana de Micología* 34, 229–232.

Scantlebury, C.E., Pinchbeck, G.L., Loughnane, P., Aklilu, N., Ashine, T. *et al.* (2016) Development and evaluation of a molecular diagnostic method for rapid

detection of *Histoplasma capsulatum* var. *farciminosum*, the causative agent of epizootic lymphangitis, in equine clinical samples. *Journal of Clinical Microbiology* 54, 2990–2999.

Secombe, C.J., Lester, G.D. and Krockenberger, M.B. (2017) Equine pulmonary cryptococcosis: a comparative literature review and evaluation of fluconazole monotherapy. *Mycopathologia* 182, 413–423.

Pythiosis

Fonseca, A.O., Botton Sde, A., Nogueira, C.E., Corrêa, B.F., Silveira Jde, S. *et al.* (2014) In vitro reproduction of the life cycle of *Pythium insidiosum* from kunkers' equine and their role in the epidemiology of pythiosis. *Mycopathologia* 177, 123–127.

Gaastra, W., Lipman, L.J., de Cock, A.W., Exel, T.K., Pegge, R.B. *et al.* (2010) *Pythium insidiosum*: an overview. *Veterinary Microbiology* 146, 1–16.

Grooters, A.M. and Gee, M.K. (2002) Development of a nested polymerase chain reaction assay for the detection and identification of *Pythium insidiosum*. *Journal of Veterinary Internal Medicine* 16, 147–152.

Mendoza, L. and Newton, J.C. (2005) Immunology and immunotherapy of the infections caused by *Pythium insidiosum*. *Medical Mycology* 43, 477–486.

Mendoza, L., Mandy, W. and Glass, R. (2003) An improved *Pythium insidiosum*-vaccine formulation with enhanced immunotherapeutic properties in horses and dogs with pythiosis. *Vaccine* 21, 2797–2804.

Pires, L., Bosco Sde, M., da Silva, N.F. Jr and Kurachi, C. (2013) Photodynamic therapy for pythiosis. *Veterinary Dermatology* 24, 130–136.e30.

Presser, J.W. and Goss, E.M. (2015) Environmental sampling reveals that *Pythium insidiosum* is ubiquitous and genetically diverse in North Central Florida. *Medical Mycology* 53, 674–683.

Rujirawat, T., Sridapan, T., Lohnoo, T., Yingyong, W., Kumsang, Y. *et al.* (2017) Single nucleotide polymorphism-based multiplex PCR for identification and genotyping of the oomycete *Pythium insidiosum* from humans, animals and the environment. *Infection, Genetics and Evolution* 54, 429–436.

Santos, C.E., Marques, L.C., Zanette, R.A., Jesus, F.P. and Santurio, J.M. (2011) Does immunotherapy protect equines from reinfection by the oomycete *Pythium insidiosum*? *Clinical and Vaccine Immunology* 18, 1397–1399.

9 Clinical Approach to Ulcerative Diseases

Erosions and ulcers are defects in the integrity of the epidermis and can occur for a multitude of reasons in horses. For example, they can develop as a consequence of severe pruritus, an ischemic insult of the skin as in the case of vasculitis or a ruptured primary lesion such as the draining of a nodule or the opening of a vesicle or bulla. In addition, any time that crusts are prematurely removed or lost, erosions can occur; therefore, erosions can also be present in pustular/crusting diseases such as *Dematophilus* infection or pemphigus foliaceus. It is thus very important to obtain an accurate history to identify the progression of the disease and the initial presence of primary lesions, which can shed light on the primary triggering cause, and to carry out a thorough physical examination to try to identify any primary lesions, which can help provide insight on the underlying disease. In the absence of this information, it can be difficult to identify the underlying disease and the clinician is left with only the secondary lesions.

It is important to note that, when biopsies are taken, the ulcerated areas should be avoided and instead a lesion that is close by and appears fresh, and that still has an intact epidermis, should be taken. Although it is often tempting to biopsy the worst-looking lesions, the answer is frequently to be found in the smaller and less impressive lesions. Many diseases require an intact epidermis for diagnosis and thus it is crucial to identify these lesions.

If the lesions are triggered by severe pruritus (Figs 9.1–9.3), the case needs to be worked up for pruritic diseases. It is important to diagnose and address the underlying disease to successfully control the pruritus, rather than relying on symptomatic therapy (see Chapter 4, this volume). For example, a severely insect-allergic horse may fail to respond to glucocorticoids if the secondary infection is not addressed and additional bites are not prevented or minimized. As a general rule, the work-up of pruritic horses relies on effective control of parasites, a reduction of insect exposure, deworming, a possible food trial and treatment of all secondary infections.

Ulcers can also be the consequence of an ischemic event, as seen in cases of vasculitis. In these cases, it is important to diagnose and control the underlying disease that triggered the vasculitis. Vasculitis can be triggered by a multitude of factors ranging from vaccines to drugs or infections, and is often precipitated by UV exposure. For example, the legs of lightly pigmented horses are frequently affected by UV-induced leukocytoclastic vasculitis in warm climates. This condition can be severe and may be accompanied by edema and extensive erosions and ulcerations in the pastern area (Fig. 9.4). Vaccines are frequently a cause of vasculitis (Figs 9.5–9.7), and reactions tend to worsen with subsequent exposures. Therefore, it is important to identify the trigger and avoid future exposures. Some cases of drug- or vaccine-induced vasculitis require short-term immunomodulation, while others may require long-term immunomodulation as the immune response can become self-sustaining. It is impossible to predict what the outcome will be other than by doing an initial course of immunomodulation and then tapering the medications to see whether a flare occurs or not. An example of vasculitis triggered by infection is purpura hemorrhagica and the most common culprit is *Streptococcus equi*, although it has also been reported in horses with *Corynebacterium pseudotuberculosis* infection. This severe necrotizing vasculitis frequently occurs after an upper respiratory infection or as a result of vaccines containing the *S. equi* M protein. In purpura hemorrhagica, vascular deposition of IgA–streptococcal M protein complexes produces ischemia and complete focal infarction of skeletal muscle and internal organs. Clinical signs can be severe and involve not just the skin but also internal organs. Purpuric lesions of the skin and mucous membranes develop, and edema of muscle and subcutaneous tissue can

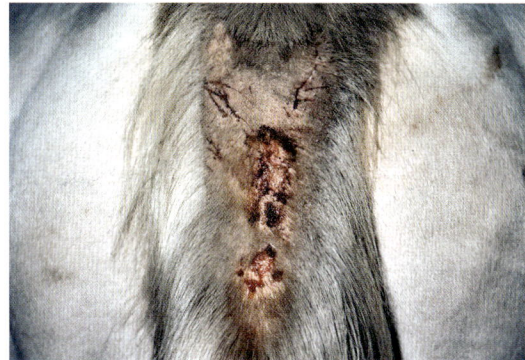

Fig. 9.1. Erosions and ulcerations on the tail of a horse with severe *Culicoides* hypersensitivity. These lesions were secondary to intense pruritus and self-trauma.

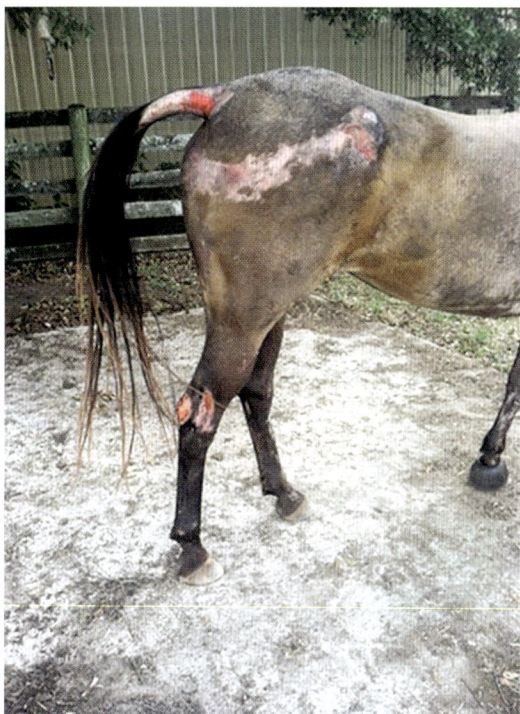

Fig. 9.2. Ulcerations on the rump, hocks and ventral aspect of the tail of a mare with a food allergy. The pruritus was unresponsive to glucocorticoids.

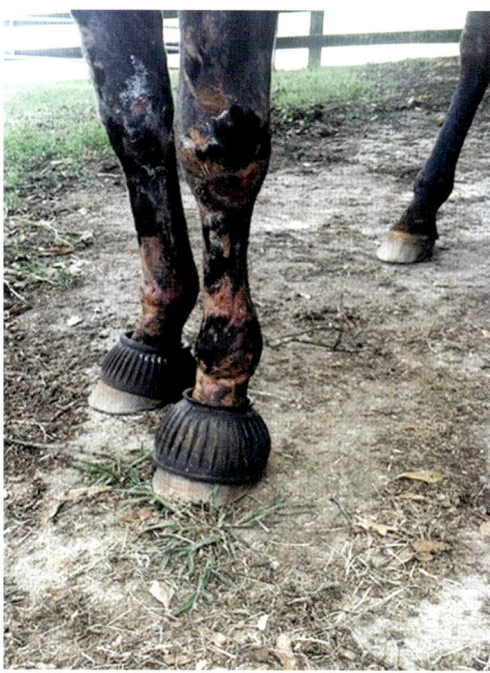

Fig. 9.3. Close-up of the ulcerations on the front leg of the horse shown in Fig. 9.2. All lesions were self-inflicted due to severe pruritus.

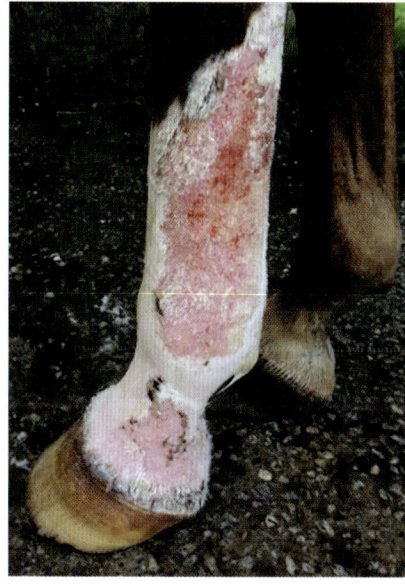

Fig. 9.4. Erosions and ulcerations secondary to UV-induced vasculitis on the non-pigmented legs of a horse. The ulcerations were the result of tissue damage and were not associated with pruritus.

follow. If thrombosis of the intestinal vessels occurs, horses can develop colic and sometimes become severely depressed. At times, fever and death can result. Prompt immunomodulation with glucocorticoids and supportive therapy are crucial in these cases.

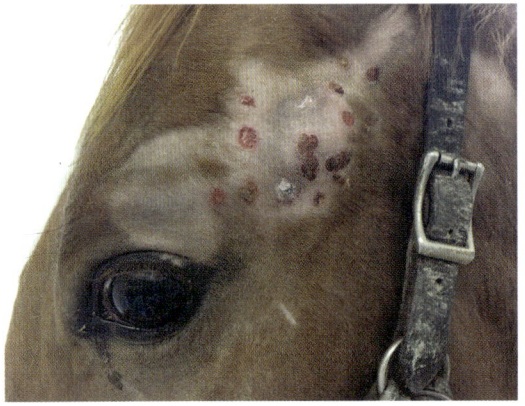

Fig. 9.5. Ulcerations secondary to vasculitis in a yearling after administration of an encephalitis vaccine. Note the circular and well-defined aspect of these ulcerative lesions. The ulcers were the result of the tissue injury associated with the vasculitis.

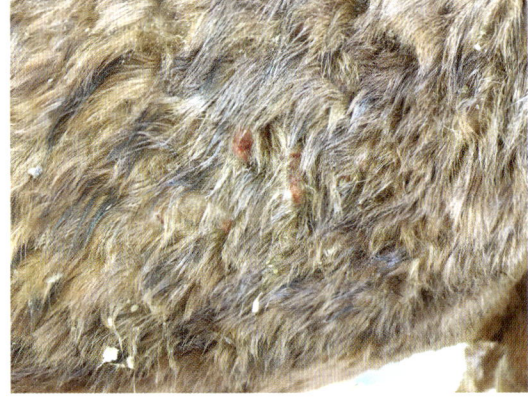

Fig. 9.7. Close-up of lesions from the horse shown in Fig. 9.5. Note the crusting and scaling. These additional lesions were due to the development of staphylococcal pustular eruptions, and rupture of the pustules has caused the scaling and the greasy seborrhea of the coat.

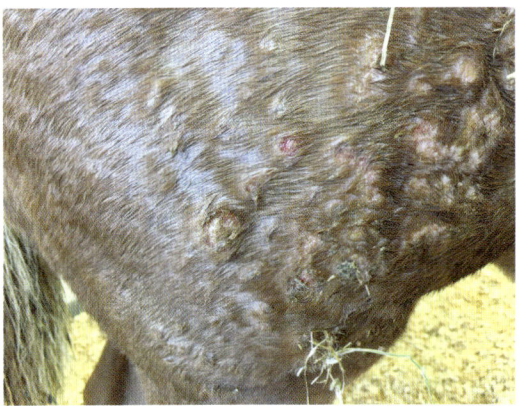

Fig. 9.6. The lateral thigh of the horse shown in Fig. 9.5. As on the face, the lesions are discrete and well circumscribed. This horse's body lesions were infected with *Staphylococcus aureus* and required an antibiotic course.

Photosensitization is another cause for the development of ulcerative lesions due to an excessive inflammatory response in the skin. This is the case in lightly pigmented horses that either ingest something that is photosensitizing (Fig. 9.8) or contract a skin infection that is photosensitizing such as dermatophilosis (Fig. 9.9), which can trigger vasculitis upon UV exposure (Figs 9.10 and 9.11). *Dermatophilus* infection can also damage the epidermis by releasing proteolytic enzymes and by inducing a massive recruitment of inflammatory

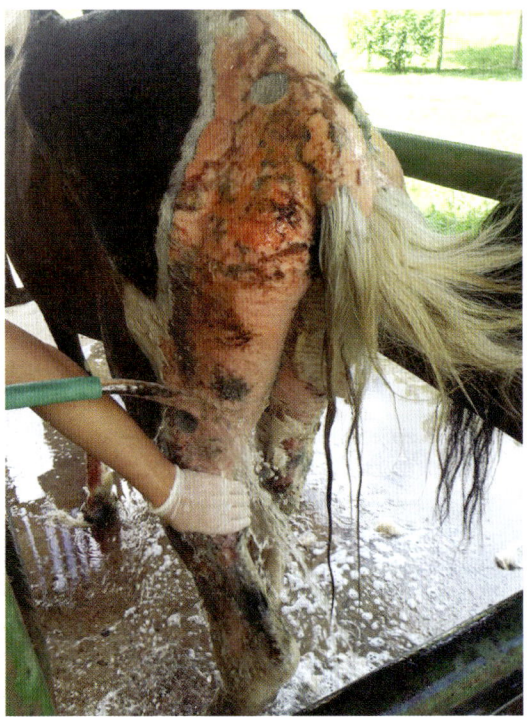

Fig. 9.8. Severe ulcerative dermatitis due to sunburn in the non-pigmented areas of a Paint horse. Photosensitization was suspected but not demonstrated.

cells such as neutrophils, which will release proteases in the skin. Therefore, ulcerations can also be seen in the absence of photosensitization when the *Dermatophilus* infection is severe. This presentation can closely mimic an autoimmune disease when seen in young foals (Figs 9.12–9.14). Therefore, it is important to examine the oral cavity to evaluate whether ulcers are present there as well. *Dermatophilus* infection is limited to the skin, while autoimmune diseases such as pemphigus vulgaris and bullous pemphigoid affect the oral cavity. Evaluation of the oral cavity allows the clinician to rank these differential diagnoses. Cytology and biopsy of affected skin that has not yet ulcerated are also important steps to achieve a correct diagnosis.

Any nodular disease where the nodules open and drain can lead to ulcerative lesions (see Chapter 8, this volume). Classic examples of nodular diseases in which ulcers are seen are habronemiasis and pythiosis. Both diseases are characterized by ulcerative hemorrhagic lesions that drain serosanguinous fluid and are extremely pruritic (Figs 9.15 and Fig. 9.16). *Habronema* has a predilection for mucous membranes, genitalia and the medial canthus of the eye (a favorite site for flies due to the moisture), while *Pythium* infection is more likely to develop on the lower legs or mouth as horses contract this disease by exposure to contaminated standing water. Although both diseases are pruritic and eosinophilic, the history and progression of the lesions are very different. Habronemiasis has a slow progression and often recurrent behavior, while pythiosis progresses rapidly and has a more acute onset.

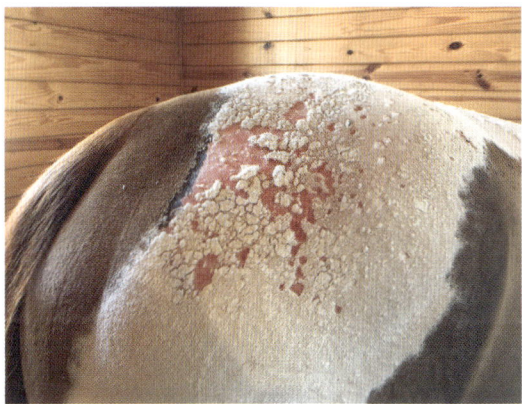

Fig. 9.9. Erosive lesions in a horse infected with *Dermatophilus*. Photosensitization in this case was linked to the infection. Note the characteristic circular lesions typical of *Dermatophilus* infection. Tenderness of the skin was noted in this horse.

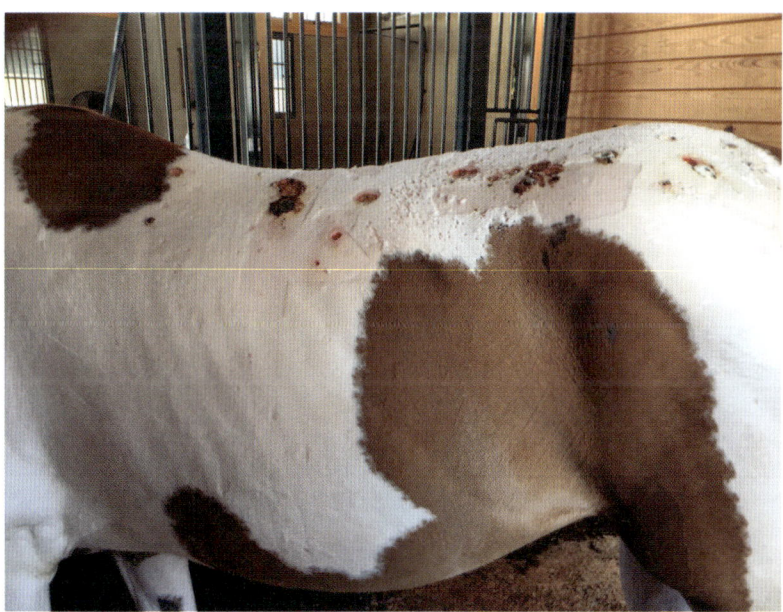

Fig. 9.10. Vasculitis secondary to *Dermatophilus* infection in the non-pigmented areas of a Paint horse. Note the sharply demarcated, deep, ulcerative lesions associated with the tissue damage caused by vasculitis.

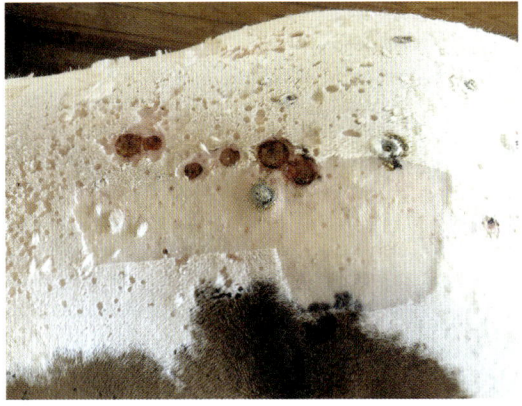

Fig. 9.11. Close-up of the vasculitic lesions of the horse shown in Fig. 9.10.

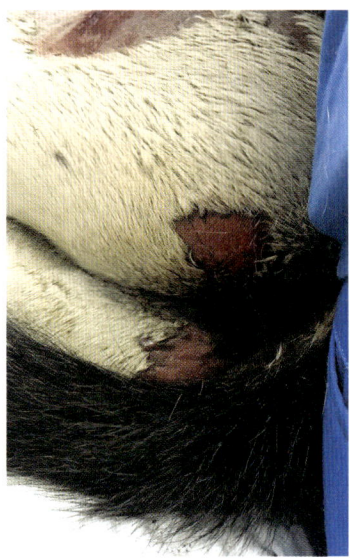

Fig. 9.13. Caudal aspect of the hind legs of the foal shown in Fig. 9.12. Ulcerative lesions had developed on areas of friction and pressure due to the release of proteolytic enzymes by *Dermatophilus*.

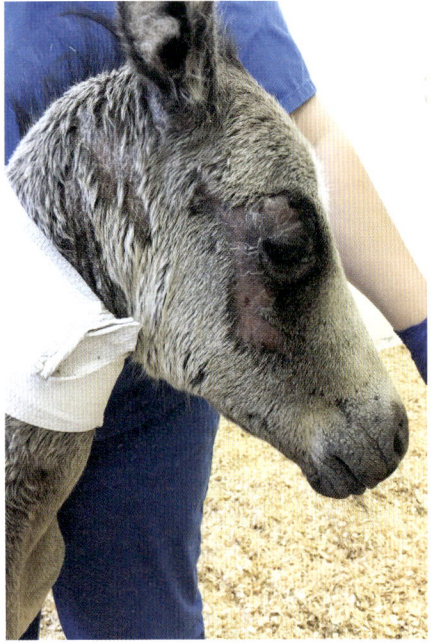

Fig. 9.12. *Dermatophilus* infection in a young foal. Note the erosive lesions around the eyes and the crusting dermatitis on the muzzle.

Diseases that present with primary lesions of vesicles and bullae are not common in horses but can occur and are primarily autoimmune disease such as bullous pemphigus and pemphigus vulgaris. These are diseases that occur in middle-aged horses when the immune system targets a component of the skin or basement membrane producing antibodies.

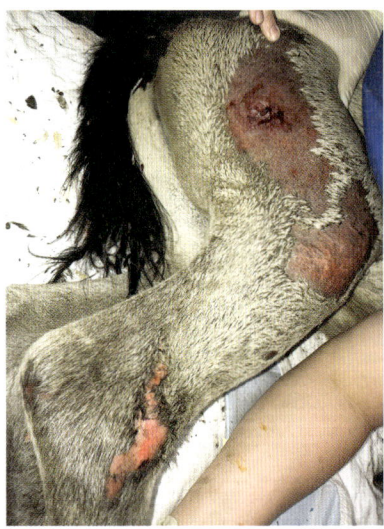

Fig. 9.14. Lateral aspect of the hind legs of the foal shown in Fig. 9.12. Pressure point areas had developed ulcerative lesions due to the severe *Dermatophilus* infection. The severe ulcerations on pressure points could have indicated an autoimmune disease in this young foal, but the absence of oral lesions and the severe *Dermatophilus* infection indicated *Dermatophilus* as the cause of these ulcerations. Complete resolution of the lesions occurred after treatment of the infection.

Most of the published information about the antigens targeted in these diseases pertains to these conditions in humans and dogs. One study in horses documented that, in equine bullous pemphigoid, IgG autoantibodies targeted the extracellular domain of collagen XVII (BP180) (Olivry *et al.*, 2000), similar to the situation reported in humans. No acantholysis is detected in cases of bullous pemphigoid. In a study of a horse with pemphigus vulgaris, it was found to have antibodies against desmoglein 3 (Winfield *et al.*, 2013). Overall, our knowledge of these diseases in horses is limited, largely due to their rare occurrence. Although the antigens targeted in these diseases are different, clinically speaking some similarities exist. The oral cavity is the first and most commonly affected site. Hypersalivation is typically present (Fig. 9.17), alerting the owner and the clinician about the presence of a problem in the oral cavity. Ulcers and vesicles are present in the oral cavity (Fig. 9.18). The skin vesicles are fragile and transient, and ulcers are the most common finding. Skin fragility and a propensity to form ulcers in areas of friction are some of the other clinical signs noted.

Diagnosis is achieved by obtaining a thorough history to rule out drug-related eruptions and a skin biopsy that shows acantholysis (in the case of pemphigus vulgaris) or subepidermal clefting (in the

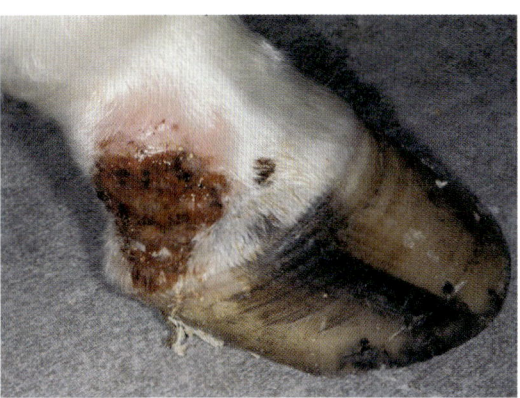

Fig. 9.15. Deep, ulcerative lesions on the pastern of a horse infected with *Habronema*. Severe pruritus was reported. A history of recurrent "summer sores" was present in this case.

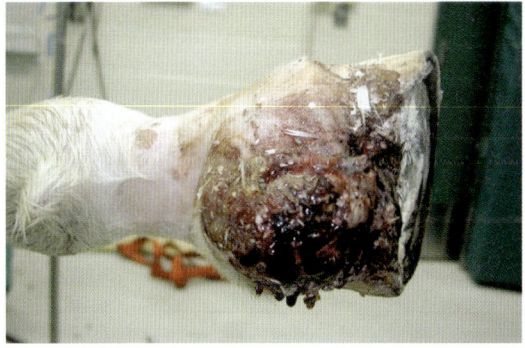

Fig. 9.16. Severe proliferative and ulcerative lesions in a horse diagnosed with *Pythium* infection. This horse had been standing in a flooded pasture after heavy rains. Rapid growth of the lesion and pruritus were the main clinical signs reported. (Photo courtesy of the Large Animal Surgery Department, University of Florida.)

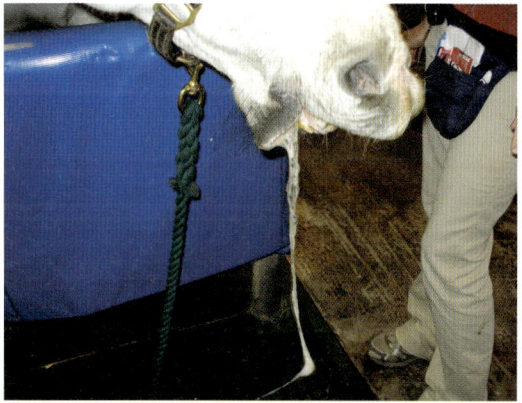

Fig. 9.17. Hypersalivation in a middle-aged horse diagnosed with bullous pemphigoid. Loss of appetite and depression were the other reported clinical signs in this case.

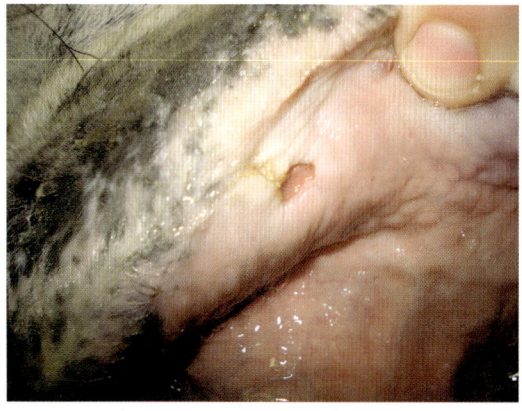

Fig. 9.18. A well-demarcated ulcer and a vesicle in the oral cavity of the horse shown in Fig. 9.17.

case of bullous pemphigoid). For both diseases, immunosuppression using high doses of glucocorticoids in combination with azathioprine can be attempted to decrease the damage to the skin. While the treatment is similar to that in pemphigus foliaceus cases, the doses of glucocorticoids required to induce and maintain remission are typically higher with pemphigus vulgaris and bullous pemphigoid, and many horses end up being euthanized due to the adverse effects of treatment (e.g. laminitis). Thus, the prognosis of these diseases is guarded to poor.

Other conditions that can present with ulcers are inherited diseases in which mutations are responsible for an abnormal basement membrane. One such disease is junctional epidermolysis bullosa, and in these cases, blistering and skin fragility are evident early on in life. In a few cases of junctional epidermolysis bullous in draft horses, the occurrence of a mutation in the laminin 5 gene has been reported, similarly to what has been reported in human Herlitz junctional epidermolysis bullosa (Milenkovic et al., 2003; Graves et al., 2009). For inherited diseases like this, there is no treatment, and affected individuals are euthanized.

An immune-mediated disease in which ulcerations and erosions can develop is erythema multiforme. This clinical syndrome can be triggered by a variety of antigens ranging from drugs to vaccines to infections. Regardless of the trigger, horses develop a variety of lesions ranging from erythematous macules to papules, urticaria-type lesions and ulcerative lesions. Some cases may spontaneously resolve, while others persist and worsen in severity. Historically erythema multiforme is characterized by scattered apoptosis of keratinocytes in the epidermis (a cytotoxic reaction), but in severe cases, it can progress to more extensive necrosis, as seen with toxic epidermal necrolysis. This syndrome, which can have the same triggers as erythema multiforme, is more severe and is characterized by full-thickness necrosis. This immune-mediated reaction can occur against drugs or other antigens that had previously been well tolerated. For successful management of these cases, it is crucial to identify the trigger and avoid it, while providing immunomodulatory drugs, such as glucocorticoids, to decrease the aberrant immune response and inflammatory response. In toxic epidermal necrolysis, the course can be rapid, and extensive areas of the skin can slough off. Depending on the extent of the areas involved, severe loss of fluids and protein can occur. Due to the impaired skin barrier function, these patients require supportive care and control of both pain and secondary bacterial infections such as *Pseudomonas*. The mortality rate of toxic epidermal necrolysis is very high in other species (as high as 90% in humans). No specific data have been published for horses. Thus, again, when presented with a case of sudden-onset ulcerative lesions, it is very important to obtain a detailed history to identify any drug, vaccine or exposure to something that could have a direct insult on the skin. Spider bites can also induce a necrotizing dermatitis that results in ulcers. Occasionally, horses may ingest caterpillars that have fallen into their feed bucket. Many of these have spines and will sting, and horses can develop significant oral ulcers that require supportive treatment.

Cantharidin toxicosis can also cause oral blisters and occurs when horses ingest alfalfa hay contaminated with "blister" beetles. The severity of the clinical signs varies depending on the amount of toxin ingested. Colic, depression and erosions of the oral mucosae are commonly reported.

Another differential diagnosis for ulcers and vesicles on the muzzle, coronary band and oral cavity is vesicular stomatitis virus (VSV) infection. This contagious rhabdovirus remains a problem in the USA, with two distinct serotypes of particular interest in this country: the New Jersey and Indiana serotypes. Outbreaks have been reported in the USA in both southern (Alabama, Georgia and South Carolina) and western (Colorado, New Mexico, Arizona, Texas and Utah) states. Affected horses can present with vesicles, ulcers, erosions or crusting on the muzzle, nares, lips, oral or nasal mucosa, tongue, ears, ventral abdomen and coronary band. Drooling and reluctance to eat are common signs. In severe cases, the skin of the tongue may slough off. When the coronary band is affected, lameness and even laminitis can develop. Horses in a pasture where no insect control is practiced are at increased risk as this virus can be transmitted by biting insects. When VSV infection is suspected, an exact diagnosis should be obtained by testing the blood for virus-specific antibodies or by testing swabs from the lesions to identify the presence of the virus. Testing is necessary to rule out the possibility that the lesions are caused by photosensitivity, irritating feeds or weeds. This is a **reportable disease** in the USA. This viral disease should not be confused with foot-and-mouth disease, which does not affect horses and which was eradicated in the USA in 1929. As there is no direct treatment for VSV, it is important to provide supportive care (e.g. soft food, proper hydration, pain control and anti-inflammatory therapy) and to minimize secondary infections. Horses can remain infective for 1 week after resolution of the lesions, and therefore it is important to isolate the horse from the rest of the herd. Regular insect control is important for prevention of this disease.

Erosions and ulcers can also be the result of direct physical, chemical or thermal injury of the skin. Examples are pressure sores as a result of ill-fitting equipment or a prolonged time on the ground, particularly in thin horses with decreased fat and muscle mass. Burns (from fires, electricity, friction or chemical exposure) will lead to ulcerations. Depending on the extent of the body that has been affected, systemic signs may be present due to loss of fluid and protein and the development of secondary infections. Supportive care and wound management are crucial for recovery. Surgical debridement, pain control, hydrotherapy and topical antibiotic administration all form part of the management. Topical silver sulfadiazine is a frequent choice in cases that can handle topical antibiotic therapy.

Severe contact dermatitis can also lead to erosions and ulcerations. Typically, this is an irritant form of contact dermatitis and is not allergic in nature. That means that the signs develop at the first exposure and elicit more pain than pruritus. All animals exposed to the same insult will develop signs. Caustic substances, bleach and iodine can all induced ulcerative lesions.

Conclusions and Take Home Messages

Ulcerative dermatitis can develop for a multitude of reasons. It is important to take a history that Home messages focuses on exposure to drugs, vaccines, other horses and specific types of hay, and on lifestyle and type of insect control, followed by a thorough examination to identify the distribution and progression of the lesions to achieve the correct diagnosis. Depending on the differential diagnoses, cytology and biopsy may be indicated. Only with proper identification of the triggering cause is it possible to implement appropriate therapy and provide an accurate prognosis to the owner. Supportive care and treatment of secondary infections is frequently needed while working up the underlying disease.

References

Graves, K.T., Henney, P.J. and Ennis, R.B. (2009) Partial deletion of the *LAMA3* gene is responsible for hereditary junctional epidermolysis bullosa in the American Saddlebred Horse. *Animal Genetics* 40, 35–41.

Milenkovic, D., Chaffaux, S., Taourit, S. and Guérin, G. (2003) A mutation in the *LAMC2* gene causes the Herlitz junctional epidermolysis bullosa (H-JEB) in two French draft horse breeds. *Genetics Selection Evolution* 35, 249–256.

Olivry, T., Borrillo, A.K., Xu, L., Dunston, S.M., Slovis, N.M. *et al.* (2000) Equine bullous pemphigoid IgG autoantibodies target linear epitopes in the NC16A ectodomain of collagen XVII (BP180, BPAG2). *Veterinary Immunology and Immunopathology* 73, 45–52.

Winfield, L.D., White, S.D., Affolter, V.K., Renier, A.C., Dawson, D. *et al.* (2013) Pemphigus vulgaris in a Welsh pony stallion: case report and demonstration of antidesmoglein autoantibodies. *Veterinary Dermatology* 24, 269-e60.

Further Reading

Duffee, L.R., Stefanovski, D., Boston, R.C. and Boyle, A.G. (2015) Predictor variables for and complications associated with *Streptococcus equi* subsp *equi* infection in horses. *Journal of the American Veterinary Medical Association* 247, 1161–1168.

Gershwin, L.J. (2018) Adverse reactions to vaccination: from anaphylaxis to autoimmunity. *Veterinary Clinics of North America: Small Animal Practice* 48, 279–290.

Olivry, T. and Linder, K.E. (2009) Dermatoses affecting desmosomes in animals: a mechanistic review of acantholytic blistering skin diseases. *Veterinary Dermatology* 20, 313–326.

Pusterla, N., Watson, J.L., Affolter, V.K., Magdesian, K.G., Wilson, W.D. and Carlson, G.P. (2003) Purpura haemorrhagica in 53 horses. *Veterinary Record* 153, 118 121.

Rodríguez, L.L. (2002) Emergence and re-emergence of vesicular stomatitis in the United States. *Virus Research* 85, 211–219.

Rosenkrantz, W. (2013) Immune-mediated dermatoses. *Veterinary Clinics of North America: Equine Practice* 29, 607–613.

Scott, D.W., Wolfe, M.J., Smith, C.A. and Lewis, R.M. (1980) The comparative pathology of non-viral bullous skin diseases in domestic animals. *Veterinary Pathology* 17, 257–281.

Spirito, F., Charlesworth, A., Linder, K., Ortonne, J.P., Baird, J. and Meneguzzi, G. (2002) Animal models for skin blistering conditions: absence of laminin 5 causes hereditary junctional mechanobullous disease in the Belgian horse. *Journal of Investigative Dermatology* 119, 684–691.

Urie, N.J., Lombard, J.E., Marshall, K.L., Digianantonio, R., Pelzel-McCluskey, A.M. *et al.* (2018) Risk factors associated with clinical signs of vesicular stomatitis and seroconversion without clinical disease in Colorado horses during the 2014 outbreak. *Preventive Veterinary Medicine* 156, 28–37.

10 Clinical Approach to Alopecia

Alopecia can result from trauma or a pathological process involving the hair follicle or the hair follicle cycle (Fig. 10.1). The vast majority of cases of alopecia in horses are pruritic and inflammatory. Bacterial folliculitis is by far the most common cause of multifocal alopecia in horses (Fig. 10.2). This can be pruritic or not. If the folliculitis progresses to rupture of the hair follicle, nodules may develop (furunculosis). If pruritus is the cause of the alopecia, the patient needs to be worked up for this as the primary presenting sign (see Chapter 4, this volume, for details).

If no history is available, examination of the tips of the hairs will provide information on whether pruritus is playing a role or not (Table 10.1). In pruritic patients, the tips will be broken and the hairs will show signs of breakage and deformity. If the hair is falling out in patches, then folliculitis should be considered as a primary problem. Causes of folliculitis in horses include *Staphylococcus*, *Dermatophilus* and dermatophyte infections. Demodicosis (caused by an abnormal proliferation of *Demodex* mites) is rather rare in horse. As the causes of folliculitis in horses also cause pustular eruption and crusting, these diseases have been discussed in detail in Chapter 7 (this volume).

If folliculitis has been ruled out or addressed, another possible cause for focal hair loss is a direct insult of the hair follicles in the area. That can be the result of an idiopathic immune-mediated process, such as in alopecia areata. In this immune-mediated disease, the bulb of hair is targeted by lymphocytes and the consequence is hair loss. This alopecia is typically non-pruritic or non-inflammatory from the clinical standpoint, even if it is inflammatory histologically, at least in the early stages. The lesions are typically on the head, although it has also been reported in other body areas. Antibodies against the hair follicles were documented in one case of alopecia areata in a horse (Tobin *et al.*, 1998). Biopsies of early lesions show cytotoxic CD8[+] lymphocytes that concentrate in the bulb of the hair. Over time, the follicles become smaller and atrophic, and in the late stages of the disease, no inflammation may be evident. A genetic predisposition exists and Appaloosa and Palomino horses appear to be over-represented. Most cases involve the hair coat (Fig. 10.3), but some cases may also have involvement of the tail and mane (Fig. 10.4), and it can be partial or complete. Some breeds of horses with sparse hairs on the tail, such as Curly and Appaloosa horses, are believed to be cases of alopecia areata. The course of this disease is varied. Milder cases may resolve spontaneously or can have a waxing and waning course. More severe cases are typically permanent. Diagnosis of this disease is confirmed by histopathology. Multiple biopsies are recommended to increase the likelihood of a diagnosis. Early lesions are more likely to be diagnostic. The response to treatment varies. In the inflammatory stage, a beneficial response may be achieved using glucocorticoids or tacrolimus topically. If the hairs are miniaturized or atrophic, no clinical benefit is achieved. Importantly, this disease is purely cosmetic and is not associated with any systemic disease.

Hair loss is sometimes due to local ischemic events. This can be the case with alopecia that occurs at the site of injections, such as vaccines or drugs. Alopecia develops over the course of several weeks and is typically permanent. A biopsy can confirm the presence of ischemic damage and vasculitis.

In other cases, hair loss may be linked to alterations in the hair cycle. The most documented in horses is anagen or telogen defluxion (also called effluvium). In the case of anagen defluxion, a stressful event interferes with the anagen growth phase and causes sudden loss of hairs within days of the event. In the case of telogen defluxion, a stressful event triggers interruption of the anagen phase of the hair and progression into the telogen phase. This results in extensive hair loss 1–3 months after the stressful event. The hair loss in

Approach to alopecia

Is the alopecia the result of pruritus or is the hair spontaneously falling out?

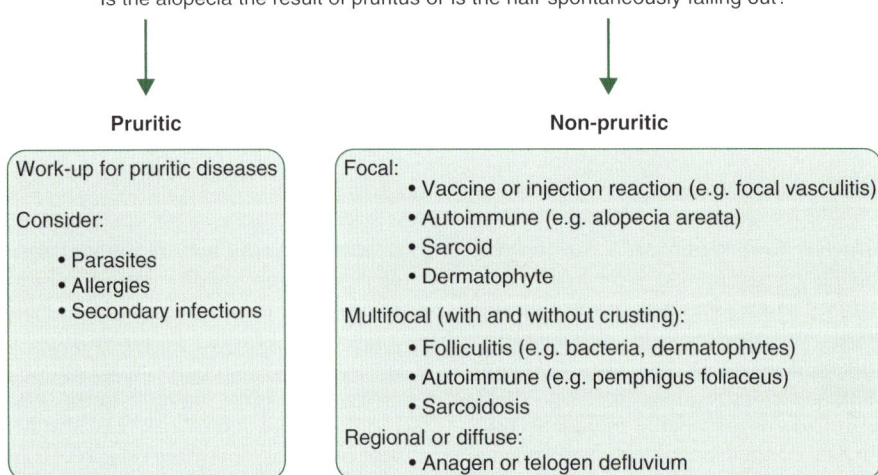

Pruritic

Work-up for pruritic diseases

Consider:

- Parasites
- Allergies
- Secondary infections

Non-pruritic

Focal:
- Vaccine or injection reaction (e.g. focal vasculitis)
- Autoimmune (e.g. alopecia areata)
- Sarcoid
- Dermatophyte

Multifocal (with and without crusting):
- Folliculitis (e.g. bacteria, dermatophytes)
- Autoimmune (e.g. pemphigus foliaceus)
- Sarcoidosis

Regional or diffuse:
- Anagen or telogen defluvium

Fig. 10.1. Common differential diagnoses for alopecia depending on presence of pruritus and the pattern of alopecia.

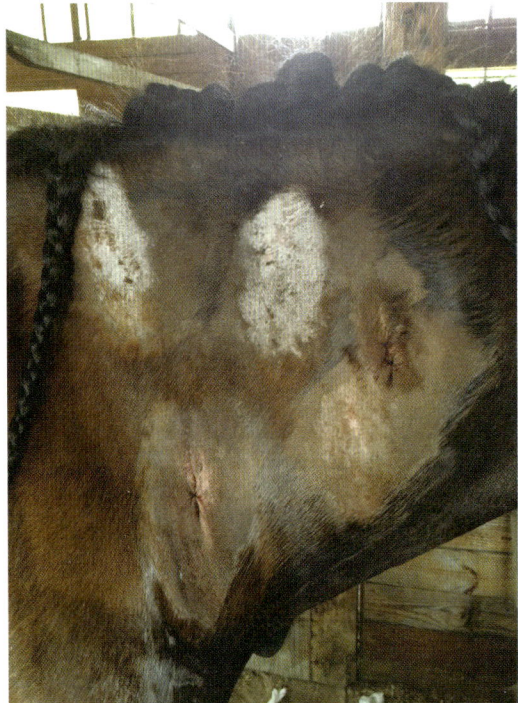

Fig. 10.2. Bacterial folliculitis leading to multifocal patches of alopecia. *Staphylococcus aureus* infection was the cause in this patient.

Table 10.1. Diagnostic work-up for a case of alopecia.

Test	Work-up
Trichogram	Check for evidence of trauma to the hair (e.g. broken tips), the stage of hair growth (anagen versus telogen) and the presence of arthrospores
Tape cytology	Check for the presence of bacteria, yeasts and inflammatory cells
Skin scraping	Check for the presence of mites
Dermatophyte test medium (DTM)	Submit a sample for culture to rule out dermatophytes
Biopsy	Based on the history and clinical signs, a biopsy may be indicated to diagnose some diseases (e.g. autoimmune, alopecia areata) once secondary infections have been cleared or ruled out

these diseases is typically more generalized and can affect larger body regions than what is seen with folliculitis (Figs 10.5–10.7). The exact mechanism of these two conditions is not well established. Hormonal changes (e.g. cortisol release) have been hypothesized to be one of the causes of the shifts in the hair cycle observed in these conditions. Another proposed mechanism for hair loss under stressful conditions involves neurotrophins, a family of growth factors that control the development, maintenance and apoptotic death of neurons, and also fulfil multiple regulatory functions outside the nervous system including hair growth. Causes for either of these defluxions are systemic disease, surgery, fever, pregnancy, cytotoxic drugs, infectious diseases and metabolic diseases. With anagen defluxion, examination of the hairs on a trichogram may show dysplastic changes with deformed and weakened hairs.

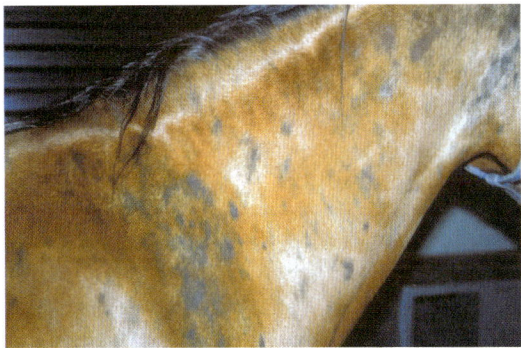

Fig. 10.3. An example of multifocal alopecia areata. It is important to rule out folliculitis before considering alopecia areata.

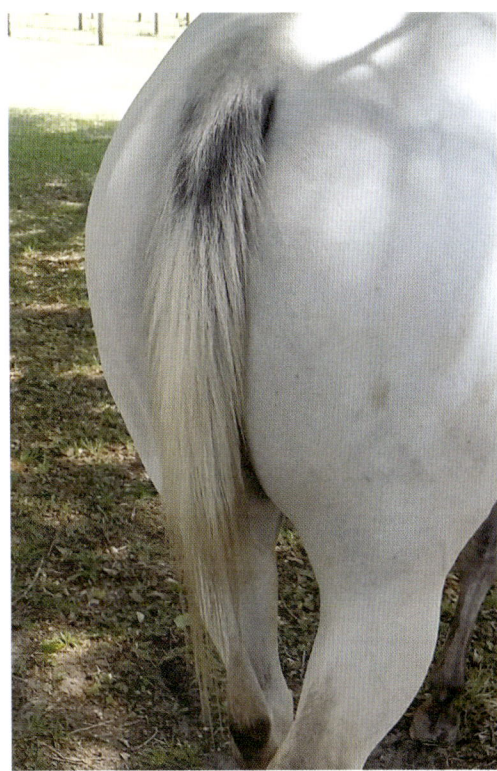

Fig. 10.4. An example of regional alopecia areata. The tail can be one area that is affected, as shown in this patient. No pruritus was present in this case.

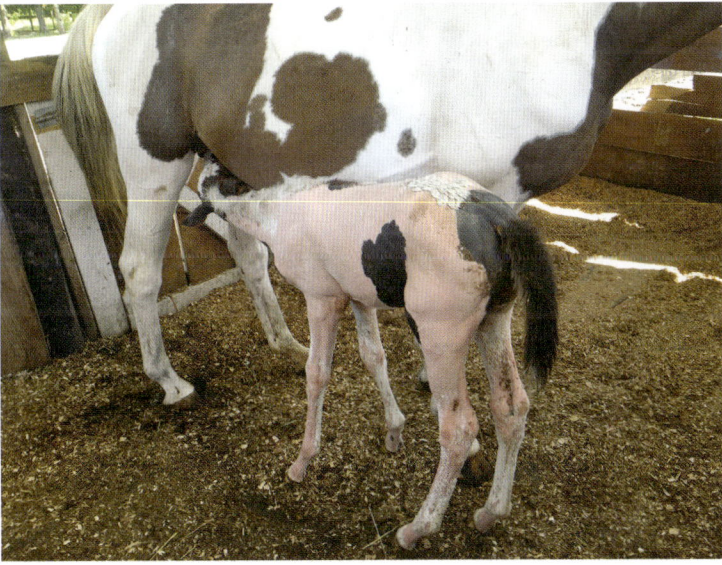

Fig. 10.5. Massive sudden-onset hair loss (telogen effluvium) in a young foal after a severe illness.

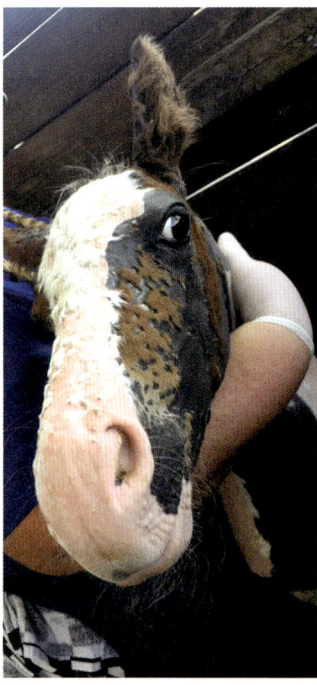

Follicular dysplasia cases have been described in horses. This can be restricted to the mane and tail, or may be limited to either black or white patches of the body. The black and tail dystrophy are now believed to be long-standing cases of alopecia areata. Rarely, dysplasia in horses may be linked to color dilution, as occurs in dogs. Regardless of these differentials, a skin biopsy is the necessary diagnostic test. There is no treatment for any of these diseases other than avoidance of trauma of the hairs as they are more fragile and more prone to secondary infections.

Rarely in horses, endocrine diseases can cause hair loss. Few cases of hypothyroidism have been described in the literature (Breuhaus, 2011). Some cases were congenital, while others were in adult horses. Thus, hypothyroidism can be considered as a differential diagnosis of hair loss, but it is not as common in horses as it is in small animals.

Finally, hair loss in horses can be due to toxicosis, such as chronic low-grade selenium toxicosis caused by ingestion of plants that concentrate selenium. Deformities of the hoof and loss of mane and tail hair are some of the symptoms of chronic toxicity.

Fig. 10.6. Close-up of the face of the foal shown in Fig. 10.5.

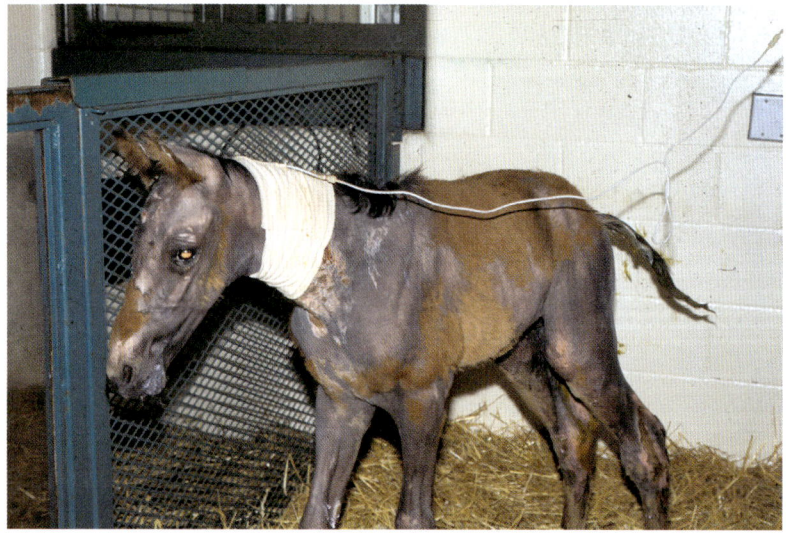

Fig. 10.7. Telogen effluvium in a young sick foal with severe diarrhea.

Conclusions and Take Home Messages

Alopecia in horses can be caused by a variety of diseases. Folliculitis and pruritic diseases are by far the most common cause. Alopecia areata or hair follicle dysplasia should be considered in cases of focal or multifocal alopecia once causes of infectious folliculitis have been ruled out. A skin biopsy is necessary to diagnose these conditions.

References

Breuhaus, B.A. (2011) Disorders of the equine thyroid gland. *Veterinary Clinics of North America: Equine Practice* 27, 115–128.

Tobin, D.J., Alhaidari, Z. and Olivry, T. (1998) Equine alopecia areata autoantibodies target multiple hair follicle antigens and may alter hair growth. A preliminary study. *Experimental Dermatology* 7, 289–297.

Further Reading

Bruet, V., Degorce-Rubiales, F., Abadie, J. and Bourdeau, P. (2008) Severe alopecia areata and onychodystrophy on all four feet of a French trotter mare. *Veterinary Record* 162, 758–760.

Colombo, S., Keen, J.A., Brownstein, D.G., Rhind, S.M., McGorum, B.C. and Hill, P.B. (2004) Alopecia areata with lymphocytic mural folliculitis affecting the isthmus in a thoroughbred mare. *Veterinary Dermatology* 15, 260–265.

Harrison, S. and Sinclair, R. (2002) Telogen effluvium. *Clinical and Experimental Dermatology* 27, 389–385.

Rosychuk, R.A. (2013) Noninflammatory, nonpruritic alopecia of horses. *Veterinary Clinics of North America: Equine Practice* 29, 629–641.

Sperling, L.C. (2001) Hair and systemic disease. *Dermatologic Clinics* 19, 711–726.

11 Clinical Approach to Pastern Dermatitis

Pastern dermatitis is a common dermatological syndrome. It is not a specific diagnosis but is a term used to describe cutaneous lesions that affect the lower legs of horses. Many diseases can induce lesions in this area, and they are frequently lumped together under this term. Slang terms for pastern dermatitis include scratches, dew poisoning, greasy heel, mud foot, mud fever, foot rot and cracked heels. All of these terms are descriptive of clinical presentations but have no diagnostic value.

When approaching a case of pastern dermatitis, it is important to consider all factors contributing to the disease. They include predisposing factors (factors that increase the risk of development of the disease but, by itself, are not sufficient to cause disease, such as the presence of feathers or prolonged exposure to mud), the primary factors (factors that by themselves can cause disease, such as *Chorioptes* or insect allergy) and the perpetuating factors (factors that prevent resolution of the disease, even when the primary cause has been removed) (Table 11.1). Examples of perpetuating factors are secondary infections.

For successful management of pastern dermatitis, it is important for the clinician to properly identify and correct all of these factors. Addressing only the secondary infection without identifying the primary cause, and vice versa, will lead to treatment failure. Regardless of the inciting cause, secondary infections are a common complication and can make the diagnostic and therapeutic process quite challenging. Therefore, it is important to have a systematic and logical approach in any case of pastern dermatitis to accurately diagnose and correct all the factors that play a role in the individual patient. It is important to address pastern dermatitis cases as early as possible, as in chronic cases it can be particularly difficult to diagnose the underlying cause.

The clinical approach starts with a thorough history including the age of onset, progression, seasonality and the lifestyle of the patient. It is important to take note of the response to previous therapies as well as the duration of treatment. It is also important to know whether the disease was treated topically or systemically, and which topical products were used. As part of the history, it is crucial to know whether the pruritus was primary (evident at the beginning) or secondary (progressive over time once the lesions and secondary infections developed). Draft horses and horses with feathers on their lower legs are prone to the development of pastern dermatitis. Thus, the presence of feathers is considered a predisposing factor for pastern dermatitis. Feathers trap moisture and allergens and so the skin underneath becomes more vulnerable to developing disease. Horses with white legs are also more prone to disease as they are at increased risk for vasculitis, which is induced by UV light. Therefore, a lack of pigment is considered another predisposing factor for pastern dermatitis.

Most horses have some level of pruritus and discomfort at the initial time of presentation. Some cases are mild and may only present with erythema, crusting and scaling (a mild form also often referred to as scratches), while others may develop significant crusting, oozing, edema (an exudative form, often referred to as greasy heel or dew poisoning) and pain. The swelling can be so severe that it leads to lameness. Chronic cases can develop severe proliferative changes. This form is often referred to as grapes or verrucous pododermatitis. Draining tracts can form, and granulation tissue formation can become significant. Lichenification, fissures and hyperpigmentation are evident in chronic cases.

On physical examination, it is important to note whether the front limbs only or all four legs are affected, and whether only depigmented limbs are involved or whether the lesions are independent of pigmentation. It is also important to know whether there are other horses affected in the herd. In many cases, the caudal aspect of the pastern is the most affected and the hind legs are affected first, although this is not always the case.

Differential diagnoses for the primary causes of pastern dermatitis are allergic (e.g. contact, atopic dermatitis, food, *Culicoides* hypersensitivity), parasitic (e.g. *Chorioptes*, *Habronema*), bacterial (e.g. *Dermatophilus*), fungal (e.g. dermatophytes), immune-mediated (e.g. vasculitis), and autoimmune (e.g. pemphigus foliaceus). As the list is extensive, it is important to address any secondary infections

Table 11.1. Some of the common primary and perpetuating factors involved in pastern dermatitis.

Predisposing factors	Genetic
	Keratinization disorders
	Exposure to a wet environment
	Feathers
	Non-pigmented pastern
Primary factors	Parasites, e.g. *Chorioptes*
	Dermatophytes
	Dermatophilus
	Allergies, e.g. contact, insects, food, atopic dermatitis
	Photosensitization
	Vasculitis
	Pemphigus
	Neoplastic, e.g. sarcoids
Perpetuating factors	Secondary infections, e.g. *Staphylococcus*, *Pseudomonas*, *Malassezia*
	Pathological skin changes, e.g. fibrosis
	Environmental factors, e.g. exposure to excessive moisture

first and treat any that are treatable, and to reassess once these infections are resolved.

The initial work-up of most cases includes skin scraping, cytology and a fungal culture (Table 11.2). A bacterial culture is frequently also recommended, particularly in chronic cases that have been treated with multiple courses of antibiotics. The best way to obtain a bacterial culture is by a skin biopsy, particularly in cases where the infection is deep. Simply swabbing the skin or a draining tract may lead to culture of secondary contaminants while missing the main pathogen. Therefore, a skin biopsy and culture of the tissue is the most appropriate way to culture these cases.

Staphylococcus is a very common cause of secondary infection. Severe cases can also be complicated by *Pseudomonas* infection as a secondary invader. Staphylococcal infections are typically treated with systemic courses of potentiated sulfonamides, although resistance is possible and should be considered in cases that do not respond to standard therapy. Systemic therapy in chronic cases is needed for extended periods of time. Topical therapy is combined with systemic therapy to speed up the resolution of the infection. Suitable topical antibacterial therapy is in the form of antiseptics (e.g. chlorhexidine, benzoyl peroxide, oxychlorine, silver sulfadiazine cream) or antibiotics (e.g. mupirocin ointment). As topicals can sometimes be irritating, it is important to monitor the lesions for any signs of worsening. It is also important to recognize when the severity of the infection is such that topical therapy alone is not sufficient and systemic therapy is necessary. Although many owners may believe that iodine is a good

Table 11.2. Diagnostic work-up of a case of pastern dermatitis

Symptoms	Work-up
Pruritic	Considered whether the pruritus is primary or secondary
Primary pruritus: consider insect allergy, contact allergy and mites	Skin scraping and treatment for *Chorioptes*
	Cytology (positive/negative culture)
	Fly control (positive/negative intradermal skin test)
	Assess likelihood of contact allergy and consider avoidance
Secondary pruritus	Treat secondary infections (empirically or based on culture) and re-evaluate
Non-pruritic	Cytology, DTM and biopsy for histopathology
	Consider possible differential diagnoses:
	• Dermatophytosis
	• Dermatophilosis
	• Pemphigus
	• Vasculitis (particularly in non-pigmented legs)

choice for topical therapy, iodine is largely ineffective and is irritating in many cases; it is therefore not recommended.

Control of insect exposure is important in many cases of pastern dermatitis that are seasonal in warm climates. This is important because some species of *Culicoides* prefer the legs as biting sites. Thus, regular use of effective repellents (see Chapter 5, this volume) is an important aspect of the management of the majority of cases of seasonal "scratches." Some horses have a combination of both insect and pollen allergy and require allergen-specific immunotherapy in combination with aggressive insect control.

During the summer, insects and moisture can also increase the risk for developing dermatophilosis. This bacterial infection can occur if the skin has been traumatized or weakened by prolonged moisture and if there is sufficient exposure to the organism. Crusting, exudation and erythema are the main clinical signs. Many horses respond to topical antimicrobial therapy. Severe cases may also require systemic antibiotic therapy, which is the same as that used for *Staphylococcus*. Indeed, many cases have a mixed infection of *Dermatophilus* and *Staphylococcus*. Keeping the skin dry and protected are important aspects of the management. Sometimes, this may require not turning out the horses until the grass is dry in the morning and keeping the pasture mowed short.

Depending on the results of initial tests, treatment for secondary infections and for *Chorioptes* may be initiated. *Chorioptes* is a common cause of pastern dermatitis, particularly in draft horses. Severe pruritus and crusting are common signs (Fig. 11.1). Diagnosis is accomplished by finding the mites on

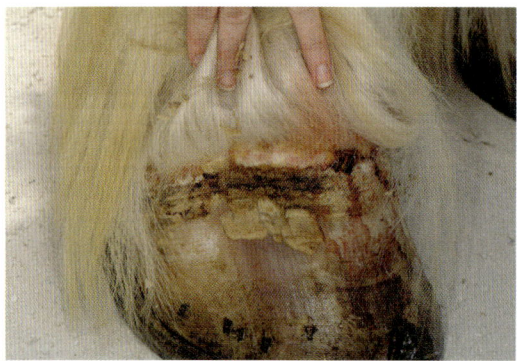

Fig. 11.1. *Chorioptes* is a common cause of pruritus and crusting, as shown in this draft horse. A skin scraping should be done in all pruritic cases of pastern dermatitis.

skin scrapings. This disease can be treated topically with lime sulfur dips (once weekly for 3–5 weeks) and systemically with ivermectin (1% solution, 0.3 mg/kg PO every 2 weeks for a total of three times) or moxidectin. Failures have been seen with this approach as the mites are very superficial and may require a topical approach rather than a systemic one (Rüfenacht *et al.*, 2011).

Shampooing with an antibacterial product (e.g. benzoyl peroxide) will help remove the crusts and can be done before the lime sulfur dip. Fipronil has also been reported to be effective, although this is an off-label use for this insecticide. It is important to note that systemic therapy may not be completely successful due to the surface habits of this mite. Topical eprinomectin has been used to successfully treat cases in which systemic treatment with oral ivermectin had failed. Other topical options to kill *Chorioptes* include topical permethrin and selenium disulfide shampoo followed by lime sulfur dips. All animals in contact with the affected animal should be treated at the same time. As the mites can survive off the host for up to 2 months, environmental decontamination is also an important aspect of treatment. Permethrin-based products can be used to spray stalls and other areas in the barn. It is also important to implement some general changes in the management of these cases. If feathers are present, it is advisable to clip the legs to facilitate topical therapy and to better visualize and clean the area. In addition, if the horses are usually kept in muddy and wet conditions, this should be changed to provide them with sufficient time in dry paddocks or clean stalls.

Many topical treatments are typically tried by owners before evaluation from a clinician, and thus it is not uncommon for patients to also have developed some form of contact dermatitis. It is therefore important only to use topical therapy that is needed and to minimize the unnecessary use of topical products that may be irritating.

Contact allergy to plants or shavings can also develop. If this is suspected, confinement can form part of the diagnostic plan. This can be done by applying bandages to the area after thorough cleaning of the skin or changing the lifestyle of the animal for 7–10 days (if no infection is present). For example, if the horse is on pasture, the animal can be stalled and only turned out in a round pen where there is no grass. If the animal is primarily in a stall with shavings, either a different type of shavings can be used or the animal can be turned out to rule out contact allergy. If a case has contact allergy that completely resolves with confinement, rechallenge should be done to confirm the diagnosis. On rechallenge, recurrence of the lesions is expected within 24–48 h after exposure. The primary lesion of a contact allergy is a pruritic papule, so horses will develop a papular eruption on the lower legs that is pruritic. Contact allergy is best managed by avoidance. If this is not feasible, then protective gear as well as oral pentoxifylline can be implemented. Pentoxifylline is dosed orally at 10 mg/kg three times daily. Allergen-specific immunotherapy is not effective for contact allergy.

If infections have been treated and allergies are not playing a role, the next step in the work-up may be a biopsy for histopathology to diagnose immune-mediated diseases such as vasculitis or pemphigus. Vasculitis is a relatively common cause of pastern dermatitis in warm climates and is frequently underdiagnosed. Cases of undiagnosed vasculitis are often presented as "resistant" cases of dew poisoning by the owner. Vasculitis can be triggered by a variety of antigens or can be idiopathic. Diagnosis of vasculitis is by biopsy. Once this is accomplished, effort should be made to identify the triggering cause, if at all possible. A careful review of drugs, dewormers and vaccinations given in the 4–6 weeks prior to the development of vasculitis should be made. Food trials can also be considered in the event that the suspected trigger is an ingredient in the horse's diet. In some cases, the disease is an immune-mediated vasculitis that appears to be aggravated by UV exposure. This disease is called photoaggravated leukocytoclastic vasculitis and particularly affects horses with white legs. This disease is believed to be caused by immune-complex deposition in the vessels of the lower legs. The vessel wall is then targeted by an inflammatory response, leading to swelling and ulcerated lesions that tend to get progressively worse and are prone to secondary infections. Thrombosis may be seen on histopathology, together with vessel wall necrosis and thickening of the vessel wall. Clinical lesions range from erythema, small ulcers and crusts (Figs 11.2 and 11.3) to larger areas of crusting (Figs 11.4 and 11.5) and ulceration, severe swelling and lameness. The lesions are more painful than pruritic. When evaluating these horses, it is important to consider photosensitization due to ingestion of photosensitizing grasses (e.g. clover, perennial rye grass, buckwheat) or other causes.

In some patients, pollens and other environmental allergens can be the triggers for the immune response in vasculitis. In these cases, it is worth

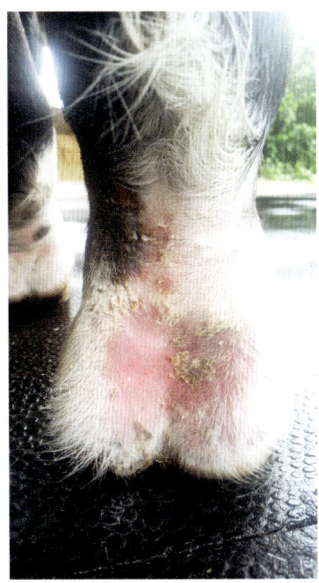

Fig. 11.2. Vasculitis is a common cause of pastern dermatitis in horses with non-pigmented legs, such as this patient. Milder cases may be confused with "scratches" and remain underdiagnosed.

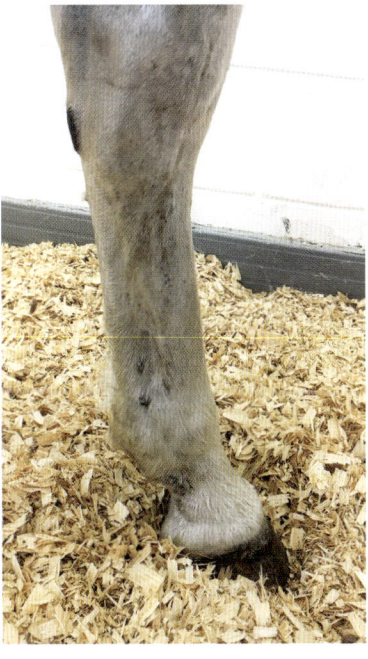

Fig. 11.3. Vasculitis in some horses leads to small, crusted lesions that become secondarily infected with *Staphylococcus*, as in this mare.

considering allergen-specific immunotherapy if the history is consistent with a seasonal problem. In the absence of the identification of a trigger, immunomodulation and protection from UV exposure are the main aspects of therapy. UV protection can be accomplished by using socks. A very effective type is silver-impregnated elastic socks (Fig. 11.6) (https://soxforhorses.com). These socks are antimicrobial and, when used daily, can lead to great improvement even after just 1 week of use (Fig. 11.7). These socks work best when kept on 24 h/day and changed daily. They are machine washable and are a good option to protect from insect bites and UV exposure.

Pentoxifylline is the drug of choice for the long-term management of vasculitis. This drug is safe for long-term use and is typically well tolerated. It has a bitter taste and can induce nervousness in some horses. It takes 3–4 weeks to achieve full effect. Glucocorticoids are frequently used to decrease inflammation at the beginning of treatment until the pentoxifylline reaches full effect. This is particularly important for moderate to severe cases that are not responsive to other treatments. In many cases, pentoxifylline and glucocorticoids are started at the same time, and after the first few weeks, the glucocorticoids are tapered off until pentoxifylline is the only drug used for the maintenance therapy. The potential for inducing laminitis should be considered before prescribing

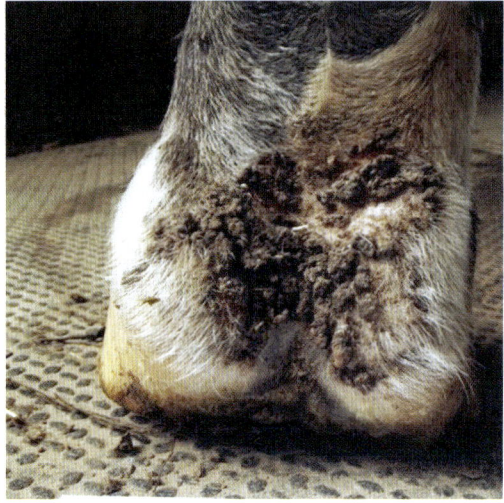

Fig. 11.4. If left untreated, vasculitis can lead to more severe crusting and ulceration, as shown in this gelding.

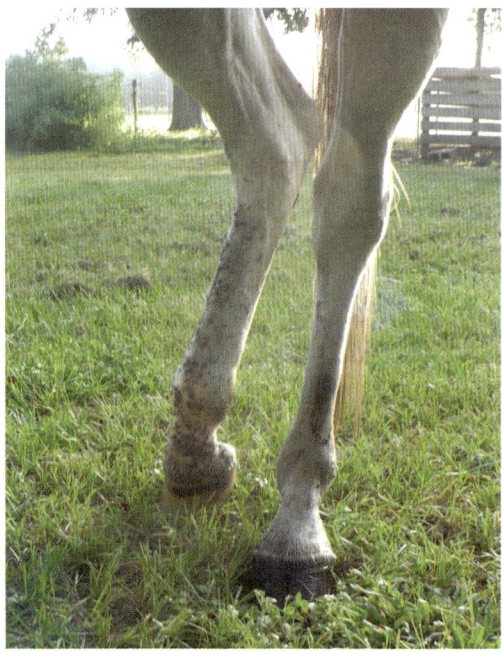

Fig. 11.5. Large areas of crusting in a horse with UV-induced vasculitis and *Culicoides* hypersensitivity.

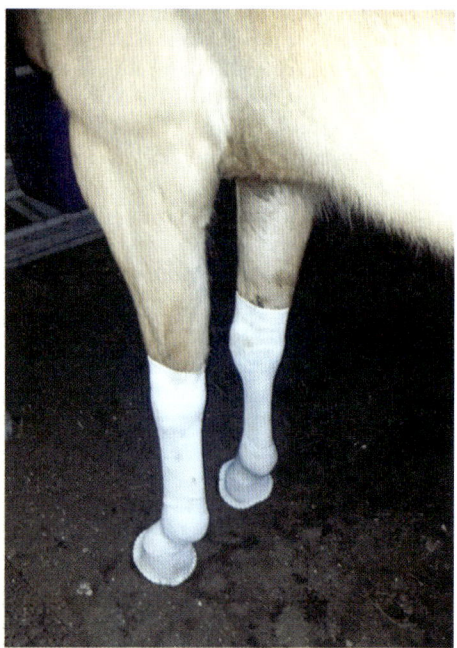

Fig. 11.6. Silver socks used by a patient with recurrent vasculitis.

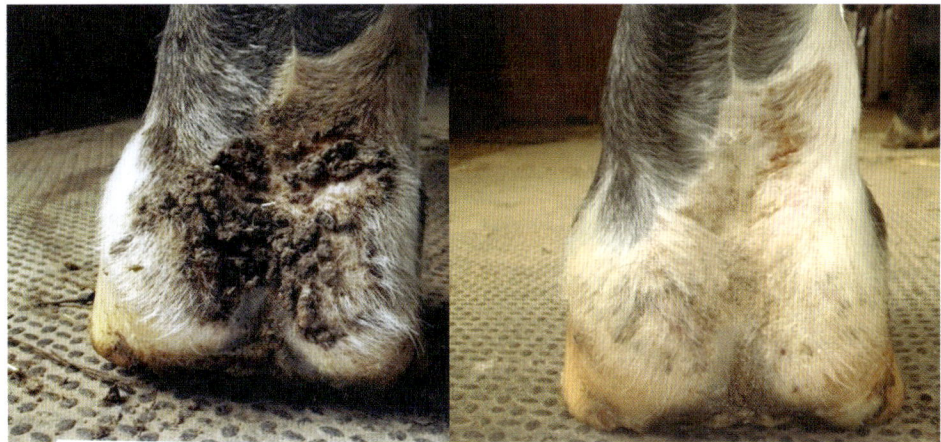

Fig. 11.7. Before and after images of a patient diagnosed with pastern dermatitis secondary to vasculitis and complicated by secondary infection. By using the socks, UV exposure was avoided and secondary infection was decreased due to the antimicrobial effect of the silver.

this form of therapy. Water therapy and mild exercise are important adjunctive strategies to decrease the swelling, particularly in horses that are stalled for extended periods of time and that tend to develop edema.

Another immune-mediated disease that can affect the pastern area is pemphigus foliaceus. In many cases, pemphigus is idiopathic and no specific trigger can be identified. In some horses, the coronary band is affected and this may be the only affected area for a long time. It is sometimes the first area affected before the disease generalizes. In pemphigus foliaceus, pustules are the primary lesions. These are transient, so are quickly replaced by areas of crusting that target the coronary band (Fig. 11.8). The disease has a waxing and waning course, and some horses may develop systemic illness at the time of a flare. Acantholytic cells can be seen on cytology. A biopsy is necessary to confirm the diagnosis. It is also important to remember that acantholytic cells may be seen in other conditions where there is a severe inflammatory infiltrate in the epidermis, such as contact allergy and dermatophytosis. For this reason, it is important to rule out dermatophytes in all cases of crusting on the lower legs of a horse. Once a diagnosis of pemphigus foliaceus is made, depending on the severity of clinical signs, the clinician will need to consider the pros and cons of treating the case with immunosuppressive drugs.

In some draft horses (Shire, Clydesdale and Belgian draft horses), a genetically inherited immune dysregulation leads to vasculitis and chronic progressive

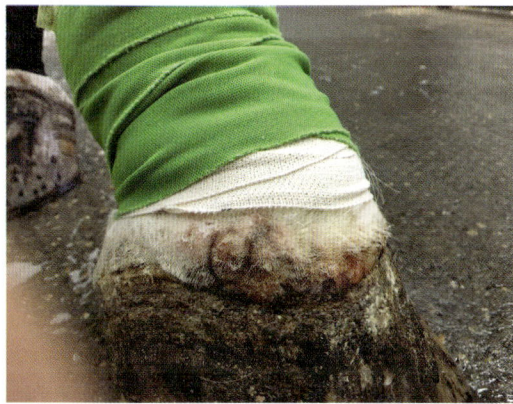

Fig. 11.8. Pemphigus foliaceus on the coronary band of a horse. In this patient, this was the only area affected.

lymphedema. This condition is characterized by progressive swelling, hyperkeratosis and fibrosis of the distal limbs (Figs 11.9 and 11.10). The disease starts at an early age, progresses throughout the life of the horse, and often ends in disfigurement and disability of the limbs. This condition is thought to have a genetic component and is chronically progressive. It is believed that a dysfunction of the lymphatic system in the skin of the lower legs leads to progressive enlargement of the vessels, which, over time, becomes permanent and can be responsible for thickening of the skin and formation of folds and nodules in the lower legs. Chronic cases can have massive formation of nodules, fibrosis and proliferative changes with disfiguration. Antibodies against elastin have been detected in affected horses. One study found that horses with clinical signs of chronic progressive lymphedema had significantly higher anti-elastin antibody levels compared with clinically normal Belgian draught horses and healthy Warmblood horses (van Brantegem *et al.*, 2007). These levels correlated with the severity of lesions. These antibodies could be used for early diagnosis of this condition and possibly to help with breeding programs to limit the breeding of individuals prone to this disease. This disease is not curable, but management can be attempted to minimize the impact on the quality of life of the horse and increase its functionality for as long as possible. As part of the management, it is useful to clip the feathers, treat any secondary infection, use pressure bandages and do water therapy. An underwater treadmill can be used to improve lymphatic drainage and circulation. Manual lymphatic drainage has been reported to provide relief and increased comfort of the horse. Diuretics are also sometimes utilized to decrease the congestion in the lower legs.

Other skin diseases that tend to affect the lower legs are habronemiasis (Figs 11.11 and 11.12) and pythiosis (Fig. 11.13). Both diseases are very pruritic and nodular. While *Habronema* infestation has a slow progression and a tendency to recur year after year (seasonal summer sores), *Pythium* infection occurs rapidly and is quickly invasive. Both diseases present with hemorrhagic nodular lesions.

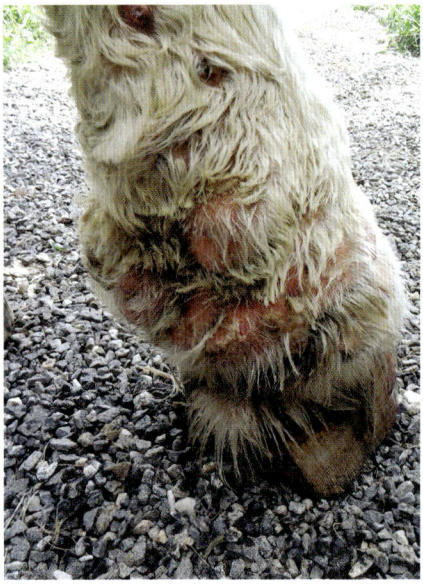

Fig. 11.9. Progressive lymphedema in a draft horse that has suffered bouts of pastern dermatitis for several years. Severe swelling and infection is present.

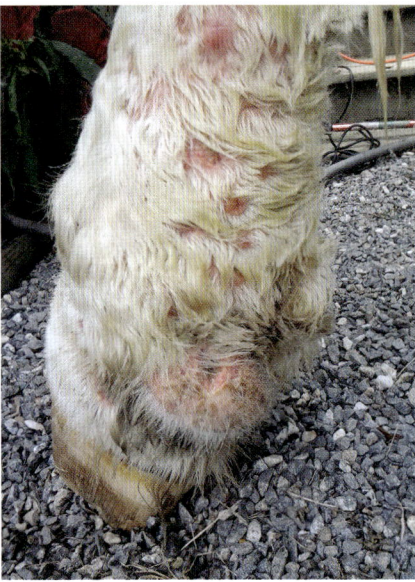

Fig. 11.10. Another leg of the horse shown in Fig. 11.9.

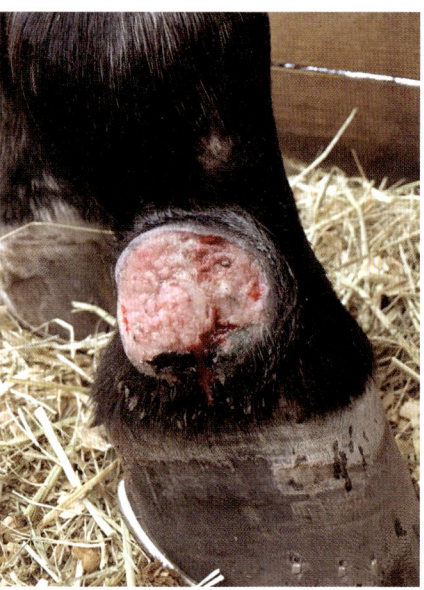

Fig. 11.11. *Habronema* infestation can cause large ulcerated nodules on the pastern of horses, as in this patient that was prone to recurrent summer sores.

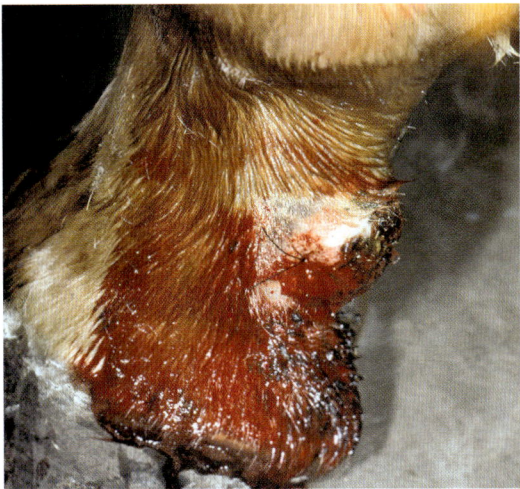

Fig. 11.12. *Habronema* infection can lead to severe pruritus and hemorrhagic lesions, as in this mare.

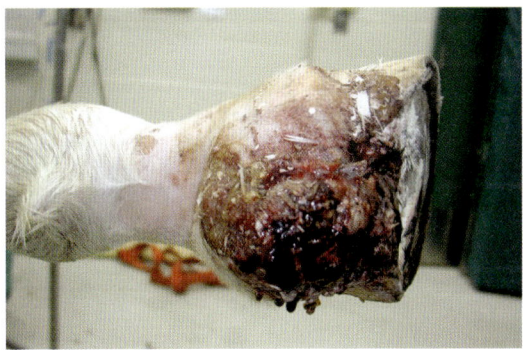

Fig. 11.13. Pythiosis can frequently affect the lower legs and lead to large nodular lesions, as in this horse that had been standing in a flooded field after heavy rains.

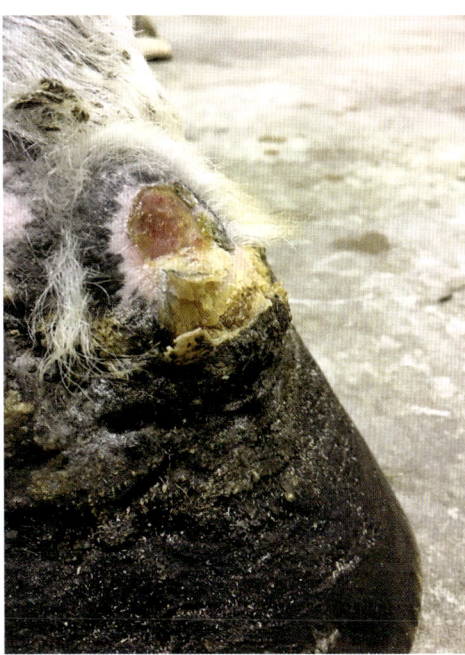

Fig. 11.14. A primary disease of keratinization with secondary infection.

On cytology, eosinophils are present in both diseases. A biopsy and special stains are helpful to diagnose pythiosis and differentiate it from habronemiasis, together with information on the clinical course. Habronemiasis is the result of a hypersensitivity reaction to the *Habronema* larvae, which are typically already dead. This is why simple deworming is typically not sufficient to provide resolution and needs to be combined with surgical debulking or a course of anti-inflammatories such as glucocorticoids, applied either to the lesion or systemically. Pythiosis requires surgical resection with wide margins, if possible. Early cases of pythiosis (less than 2 weeks' duration) also respond to immunotherapy to switch the immune response to the organisms from a humoral and Th2-type response to a cell-mediated, Th1-type response.

In cases of crusting of the coronary band that have been ongoing for some time, and when only one horse in the herd is affected, a primary disease of keratinization may be a possibility (Fig. 11.14). In these cases, increased speed of proliferation of the epidermis together with decreased desquamation leads to accumulation of a thick crust, particularly in the coronary band area (Fig. 11.15). These lesions can become infected and have proliferative granulomatous tissue due to chronic bouts of infection. A skin biopsy is necessary for diagnosis. As these cases are genetically inherited, control of the infections and the excessive crusting is the main strategy for treatment. Management is possible but a cure is not achieved. Application of keratolytic agents, such as urea, helps to loosens the crusts and slow down the proliferation of the epidermis in the area. Control of secondary infections is an important part of management.

Conclusion and Take Home Messages

Many different diseases can manifest as pastern dermatitis. Due to the numerous possible underlying causes, a systematic and logical approach is crucial.

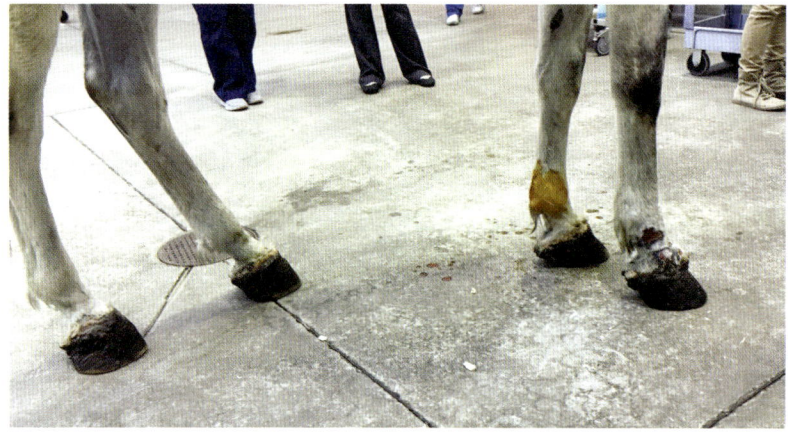

Fig. 11.15. Crusting and deformity present on the coronary band of all four feet of the patient shown in Fig. 11.14.

Taking a thorough history, careful physical examination and identification of primary lesions (when still present) are important in aiding the clinician to formulate the best diagnostic plan for each individual case. In most cases, secondary infections are present and complicate the evaluation, and thus successful identification of the underlying disease will also depend on complete resolution of the secondary infections. Many cases require topical therapy together with management changes such as the use of bandages (as long as they are changed frequently and kept dry), avoidance of muddy areas and clipping of feathers. Identification of all factors contributing to the syndrome is crucial for complete success in the management of pastern dermatitis.

References

Rüfenacht, S., Roosje, P.J., Sager, H., Doherr, M.G., Straub, R. *et al*. (2011) Combined moxidectin and environmental therapy do not eliminate *Chorioptes bovis* infestation in heavily feathered horses. *Veterinary Dermatology* 22, 17–23.

van Brantegem, L., de Cock, H.E., Affolter, V.K., Duchateau, L., Hoogewijs, M.K. *et al*. (2007) Antibodies to elastin peptides in sera of Belgian Draught horses with chronic progressive lymphoedema. *Equine Veterinary Journal* 39, 418–421.

Further Reading

Aufox, E.E., Frank, L.A., May, E.R. and Kania, S.A. (2018) The prevalence of *Dermatophilus congolensis* in horses with pastern dermatitis using PCR to diagnose infection in a population of horses in southern USA. *Veterinary Dermatology* 29, 435–e144.

Geburek, F., Deegen, E., Hewicker-Trautwein, M. and Ohnesorge, B. (2005) Verrucous pastern dermatitis syndrome in heavy draught horses. Part II: Clinical findings. *Deutsche Tierärztliche Wochenschrift* 112, 243–251.

Mittmann, E.H., Mömke, S. and Distl, O. (2010) Whole-genome scan identifies quantitative trait loci for chronic pastern dermatitis in German draft horses. *Mammalian Genome* 21, 95–103.

Poore, L.A., Else, R.W. and Licka, T.L. (2012) The clinical presentation and surgical treatment of verrucous dermatitis lesions in a draught horse. *Veterinary Dermatology* 23, 71.e17.

Psalla, D., Rüfenacht, S., Stoffel, M.H., Chiers, K., Gaschen, V. *et al*. (2013) Equine pastern vasculitis: a clinical and histopathological study. *Veterinary Journal* 198, 524–530.

Risberg, A.I., Webb, C.B., Cooley, A.J., Peek, S.F. and Darien, B.J. (2005) Leucocytoclastic vasculitis associated with *Staphylococcus intermedius* in the pastern of a horse. *Veterinary Record* 156, 740–743.

Yu, A.A. (2013) Equine pastern dermatitis. *Veterinary Clinics of North America: Equine Practice* 29, 577–588.

12 Clinical Approach to Pigmentary Changes

The color of the skin and coat depend on many factors. One of the most important is the pigment melanin, synthesized by melanocytes in both the skin and the hair. Others include blood flow, the thickness of epidermis and transmission of light. Melanocytes are derived from the neural crest, and in the skin they are located in the basal cell layer. It is important to note that, on histopathology, melanocytes actually appear as clear cells, and the dark cells seen in the epidermis on regular histopathology are not melanocytes but keratinocytes. Melanin produced by the melanocytes is transferred to nearby keratinocytes so that they appear pigmented on histopathology. Each melanocyte with its satellite of keratinocytes is known as an epidermal melanin unit. One melanocyte can supply anywhere from ten to 40 keratinocytes with pigment. The enzyme tyrosinase is important in two early and one late steps in the formation of melanin.

The skin has limited ways to react to insults, and a change in pigmentation is one way in which it can react to inflammation or trauma. The purpose of this chapter is to present a diagnostic approach to pigmentary changes in the skin and hairs of horses to help clinicians presented with horses with such changes.

Hyperpigmentation

Some of the factors affecting pigmentation are shown in Table 12.1. Hyperpigmentation can affect the skin or hair. Clinically speaking, in most cases, skin hyperpigmentation occurs as a result of chronic trauma or inflammation. In these cases, hyperpigmentation is typically accompanied by lichenification (increased thickness of the skin) as shown in Fig. 12.1. Such cases need to be worked up for chronic causes of pruritus or inflammation. Sometimes, inflammation can lead to both hyperpigmentation and depigmentation in the same individual, depending on the depth of skin damage (more superficial

trauma stimulates hyperpigmentation, while damage that extends to the basement area can lead to loss of pigment; Fig. 12.2).

Lentigo is another manifestation of hyperpigmentation, but in this case the skin does not appear thicker. In this condition, which is rare in horses, discrete hyperpigmented macules are noted. The lesions are flat, asymptomatic and non-inflammatory, and they are a cosmetic problem only. These lesions are different in appearance from melanomas, which are raised infiltrated lesions that are common in older gray horses. Although a thorough discussion of skin tumors is beyond the scope of this book, it is important to highlight that melanomas in gray horses are not associated with UV exposure, as occurs in humans, but are linked with genetic mutations of gray horses. Many of these horses also have vitiligo-like lesions (depigmented macules). Benign melanomas of gray horses are most commonly observed in the tail and perineal area. While most melanomas have a benign clinical course and slowly increase in size and number with age, they can occasionally metastasize to internal organs and have a more malignant clinical course.

Hypopigmentation

Several factors can decrease pigmentation, as shown in Table 12.1. Depigmentation can affect the skin (leukoderma) and/or the hair (leukotrichia).

Depigmentation can be genetically inherited or acquired. Albinism is transmitted as an autosomal-recessive trait. In horses, most albinos have a lack of tyrosinase, so even if melanocytes are present, they are not able to produce melanin. This affects the skin as well as the eyes.

In Waardenburg–Klein syndrome, the issue is defective migration of the melanocytes rather than production of melanin. In these individuals, melanocytes are not detected on a skin biopsy. The animals are deaf, as melanocytes have not migrated

Table 12.1. Common factors affecting pigmentation that can be used to help with the formulation of a differential diagnosis.

Category	Factors that increase pigmentation	Factors that decrease pigmentation
Hormonal	Melanocyte-stimulating hormones (α-MSH, β-MSH and γ-MSH) derived from the pituitary gland and causing activation and synthesis of tyrosinase; they are also associated with dispersal of melanosomes	Melatonin, from the pineal gland: antagonist of MSH
	Adrenocorticotropic hormone (ACTH): in patients with pituitary hyperadrenocorticism, excess levels of ACTH are produced, resulting in excessive pigmentation	Corticosteroids
	Androgens, estrogens and progesterones	
Chemical		Excessive molybdenum
		Copper deficiency (which affects tyrosinase activity as copper is a coenzyme for tyrosinase)
Genetic		Several genetic diseases can decrease pigmentation; some are lethal, while others are not. Two benign examples are: albinism (some albinos have tyrosinase deficiencies, while others have tyrosinase but produce abnormal melanosomes, known as tyrosinase-negative and -positive albinos, respectively); and piebaldism (absence of melanocytes in certain regions secondary to abnormalities in melanocyte migration and development)
Miscellaneous	UV light: stimulates activation of tyrosinase, especially UVB light (290–320 nm)	Physical destruction of melanocytes through injury, e.g. cryosurgery, freeze branding or inflammation (e.g. *Onchocerca* infection)
	Inflammation: probably mediated by prostaglandins and arachidonic acid and its metabolites	Immune-mediated destruction of melanocytes or tyrosinase (e.g. vitiligo)
	Friction: the skin becomes thicker and darker in areas of chronic pruritus and self-trauma that does not extend to the basement membrane area	Any damage to the basement membrane can lead to "pigmentary incontinence" and resulting leukoderma, e.g. lupus-type diseases or inflammation that targets the epidermal–dermal junction

to the inner ear, where they play as essential role in normal function of the ear. This is a dominant trait and is seen primarily in American Paint horses.

While these two genetically inherited conditions are not lethal, some genetically inherited diseases linked to pigmentation can sometimes be lethal. This is the case for lethal white foal syndrome. This is a recessively inherited condition and is linked to a mutation of the endothelin receptor B, which is critical for the development and migration of neural crest cells to form both melanocytes and enteric neurons. Affected horses not only lack pigmentation but also show the absence of myenteric plexuses and are unable to pass feces. Within

a short time after birth, they show signs of colic and require euthanasia as there is no treatment for this disease.

When acquired skin depigmentation is noticed, it may be due to a direct insult, an autoimmune attack of the melanocytes, the inability to produce pigment or damage of the basement membrane, leading to a decreased level of pigment in the dermis (called "pigmentary incontinence"). Damage of the basement membrane may be caused by direct attack of the membrane as seen in autoimmune diseases such as lupus, extensive inflammation in the dermis (Fig. 12.3), inflammation specifically targeting the dermal/epidermal area as in erythema

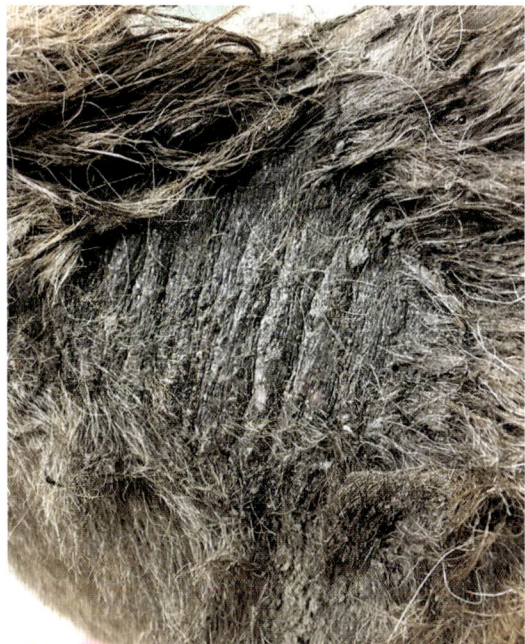

Fig. 12.1. Increased thickness and pigmentation is a common consequence of chronic trauma and inflammation, as in this case of chronic foliaceus.

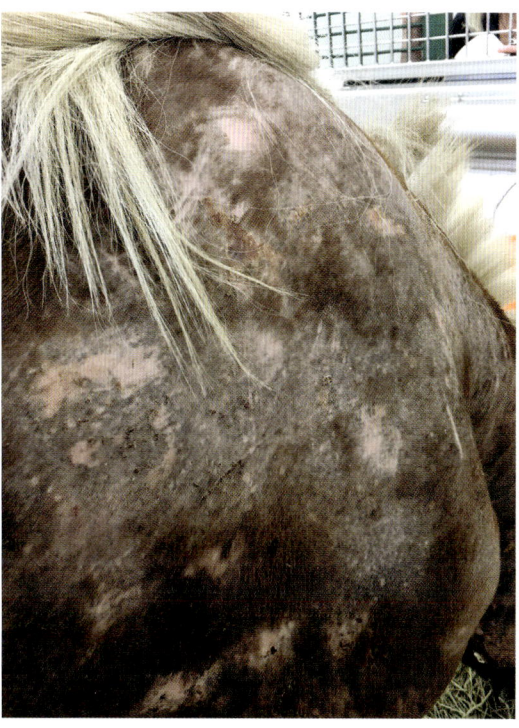

Fig. 12.2. Depigmentation is sometimes mixed with areas of hyperpigmentation, as in this chronic severe case of insect allergy. Depigmentation occurs when the skin damage has at some point extended past the basement membrane, leading to loss of pigment.

multiforme, or neoplastic accumulation of cells as in mycosis fungoides.

Three peculiar conditions in horses associated with leukotrichia are reticulated leukotrichia, spotted leukotrichia and hyperesthetic leukotrichia.

Reticulated leukotrichia appears to be genetically inherited as it is more commonly observed in Quarter horses and Thoroughbreds. The author has seen it in a family of Warmbloods crossed with Namibian horses (Figs 12.4–12.6). Whitening of the hairs in stripes and a reticulated pattern are seen on the dorsum and start in young horses. Occasionally, crusts are seen before the change of hair color. Once the crusts fall off, the hair grows in a different color. It has been proposed that this may be an unusual form of erythema multiforme, possibly linked to vaccinations. This condition is not painful, and this is the main difference from the hyperesthetic leukotrichia.

Spotted leukotrichia has been reported primarily in Arabian horses, although it can occur in other breeds as well. This condition appears to be asymptomatic in the sense that the spots develop without prior skin lesions and can be associated with leukoderma. The spots sometimes show a waxing and waning behavior and may be permanent. They are typically on the sides and rump. They are not painful or pruritic.

Hyperesthetic leukotrichia is a rare condition that is also proposed to be an unusual form of erythema multiforme. This disease affects mature horses and is painful. Horses react violently when the affected skin is touched. The whitening of the hair is preceded by crusty vesicles. The pain typically subsides once the skin lesions have gone away. Vaccination and deworming have been reported weeks to months before the development of these lesions. Recurrences have been reported. There is currently no treatment for this condition. The histopathology of these lesions is most consistent with erythema multiforme, with the special finding of large stellate CD18[+] cells, which have been proposed to be histiocytic in origin. A link with a herpes virus has been proposed due to the pain, similar to the experience of humans with herpes zoster, but negative results

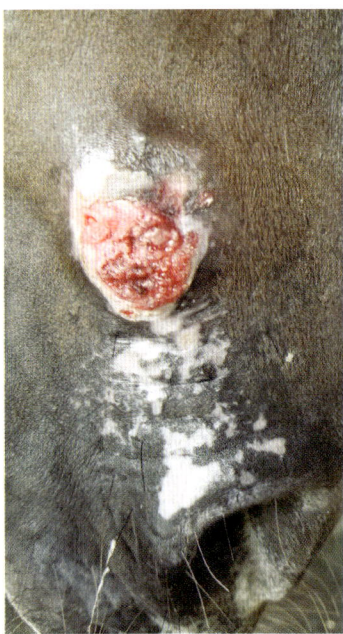

Fig. 12.3. Depigmentation as a result of severe skin inflammation and damage.

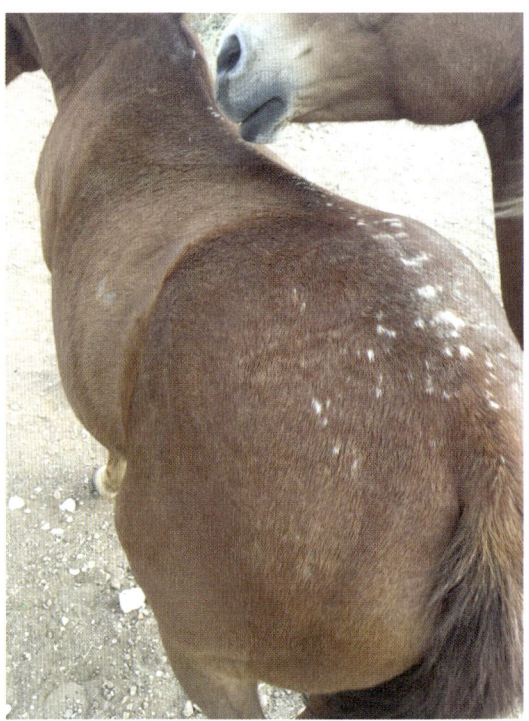

Fig. 12.5. Reticulated leukotrichia in a sibling of the horse shown in Fig. 12.4.

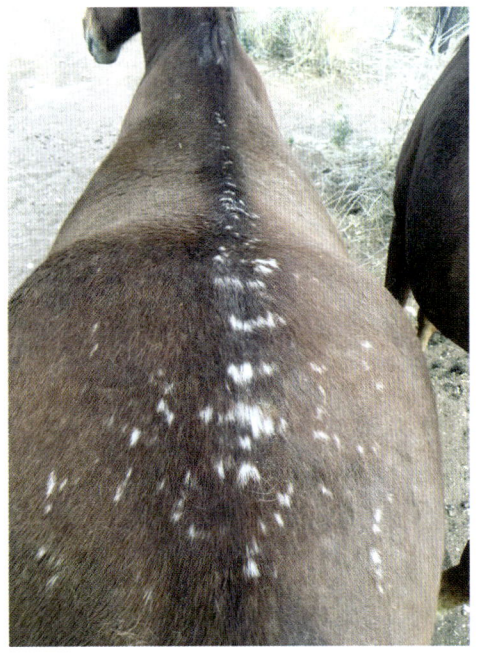

Fig. 12.4. Reticulated leukotrichia in a Namibian horse. No pain or pruritus was present in this horse.

were reported in the few horses tested and thus the reason for the pain is currently unknown.

A common cause of depigmented macules in gray horses is vitiligo. The most common theory on why vitiligo develops is an immune-mediated attack of the melanocytes. This condition has a strong genetic component and some breeds are prone to it. The depigmentation is not associated with inflammation and can affect both skin and hair. It is now known that increased melanocortin-1 receptor signaling promotes melanoma development in gray horses and it is speculated that the vitiligo lesions are caused by antibodies against melanocytes as a reaction against the melanoma (Fig. 12.7). In some gray horses, vitiligo is noticed despite no clear evidence of a cutaneous melanoma.

Melanocytes may be damaged by chemicals or may not be able to produce pigment due to enzymatic deficiencies or deficiencies of cofactors such as copper. In many benign cases, depigmentation is post-inflammatory (Fig. 12.8). Depending on the severity of the insult, this can be temporary or permanent (as in the case of branding).

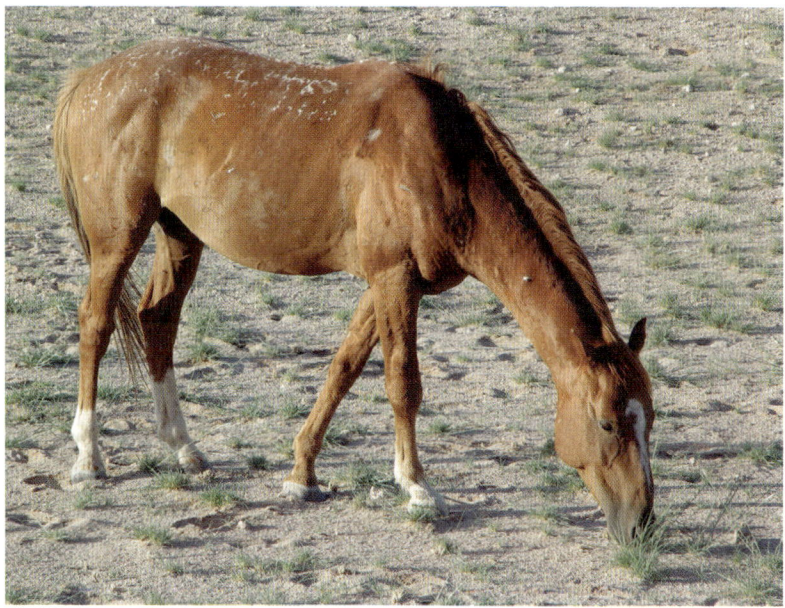

Fig. 12.6. Reticulated leukotrichia in a Namibian horse in the same herd as the horses shown in Figs 12.4 and 12.5. None of the horses had any history of pain prior to the development of leukotrichia.

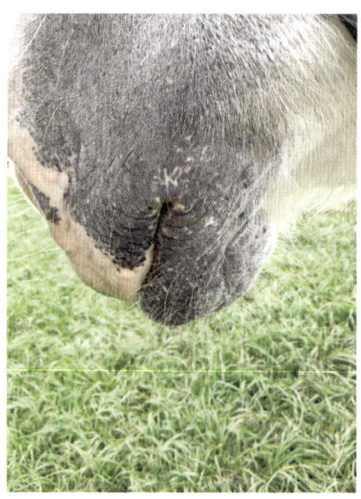

Fig. 12.7. Vitiligo in a gray horse with melanoma.

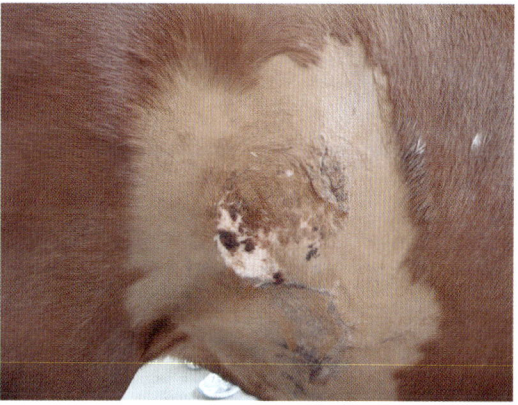

Fig. 12.8. Scarring and depigmentation in a horse recovering from a deep pyoderma.

Further Reading

Fadok, V.A. (1995) Update on four unusual equine dermatoses. *Veterinary Clinics of North America: Equine Practice* 11, 105–110.

Goodale, E.C., White, S.D., Outerbridge, C.A., Everett, A.D. and Affolter, V.K. (2016) A retrospective review of hyperaesthetic leucotrichia in horses in the USA. *Veterinary Dermatology* 27, 294-e72.

Rosengren Pielberg, G., Golovko, A., Sundström, E., Curik, I., Lennartsson, J. *et al.* (2008) A *cis*-acting regulatory mutation causes premature hair graying and susceptibility to melanoma in the horse. *Nature Genetics* 40, 1004–1009.

Useful Terms

Abrasion Superficial removal of the epidermis resulting in oozing and crusting. This is a superficial defect of the skin that does not go beyond the basement membrane.

Abscess A localized collection of pus in a cavity formed by disintegration of tissue.

Acantholysis Detachment of cells within the stratum spinosum from one another.

Acanthosis Hyperplastic thickening of the stratum spinosum (and thus the epidermis).

Adnexa Appendages of the epidermis, including hair follicles, sebaceous glands, sweat glands, mammary glands, nails, claws, hooves and hair.

Alopecia A decrease in the amount or absence of hair.

Anhidrosis A deficiency of sweating.

Blister A common term for a vesicle or bulla.

Callus Hypertrophy of the stratum corneum in a localized area of increased trauma.

Cellulitis Diffuse inflammation of the deep dermis and subcutis.

Comedo (pl. comedones) Accumulation of keratin and dried sebum in a hair follicle.

Cyst A sac that contains liquid or semi-solid material.

Dermatitis Inflammation of the skin.

Dermatomycosis A fungal infection of keratinized epidermis and adnexae (usually dermatophytosis).

Dermatophytosis Infection with *Microsporum* or *Trichophyton* spp.

Dermatosis An abnormal condition or disease of the skin.

Diffuse Not definitively limited or localized; widely distributed.

Ecchymosis Extravasation of blood into tissue spaces.

Erosion An ulcer that goes to the depth of the basement membrane.

Erythema Redness produced by capillary congestion.

Exfoliation Peeling off in scales or layers.

Exudation The escape of fluid, cells and cellular debris from blood vessels and their deposition in or on tissues; it is usually the result of inflammation.

Fissure A deep linear defect in the epidermis.

Folliculitis Inflammation of hair follicles and associated adnexae.

Furunculosis A process in which the integrity of the follicle wall has been compromised. Once a follicle ruptures, keratin can be released in the dermis triggering a foreign body reaction. A furuncle is a follicular abscess or ruptured folliculitis.

Hypertrichosis An increased amount of hair; usually due to increased length (hirsutism).

Hypotrichosis The presence of a less than normal amount of hair.

Leukoderma Decreased pigmentation of the skin.

Leukotrichia Decreased pigmentation of the hair.

Papilloma A lobulated benign epithelial tumor; usually viral.

Parakeratosis A histological term used to describe an increase in thickness of the stratum corneum in which the nucleus is still visible in the keratinized cells. This is a sign of increased speed of keratinization.

Patch A macule that is greater than 2 cm in diameter.

Pruritus Itching.

Seborrhea A functional disturbance of sebaceous glands or of lipid metabolism of the epidermis. It is accompanied by abnormal keratinization.

Serpiginous Creeping; this refers to lesions that enlarge slowly in the shape of a crawling snake.

Spongiosis Intercellular epidermal edema.

Stratum basale The innermost layer of the epidermis composed of columnar cells arranged on a basement membrane. This is the germinative layer of the skin.

Stratum corneum The outermost layer of the epidermis composed of dead keratinized epidermal cells.

Stratum granulosum A layer of the epidermis composed of flattened cells with pyknotic nuclei and keratin granules.

Subcorneal Below the stratum corneum.

Urticaria Superficial dermal edema and erythema, with circumscribed and multiple eruption of wheals.

Verrucous Wart-like.

Vitiligo Patchy change of skin pigmentation.

Index

Note: Page numbers in **bold** type refer to **figures**
Page numbers in *italic* type refer to *tables*

eumycotic mycetoma 88
excoriations 8, **10**
eyes 54, **54**

face 54, **55**
fans 37
fatty acids 20, 38
feathers 110, 118
fibrosis, distal limbs 115
fipronil 49, 112
fissures 110
Fite Faraco 14
flaxseed 22, 38
fluconazole 24, 84, 85
fluorinated steroids 20
fluoroquinolones 23, 61
fly (flies) 47, 93
 control 32, 36, 40, 47, 57
 masks 37, 47, 64, **65**
 repellents 46–47
 sheets 37, 47
 sprays 3, 20, 41, **41**
follicular dysplasia 108
follicular pustules 59
folliculitis 3, 11, 105
 bacterial 37, 40, 105, **106**
  staphylococcal 34, **36**, 38, 59–62, 79
  Streptococcus 89
 clinical signs 60
 Demodex equi 50
food
 allergy 13, 16, 40–41
  ulcers 96, **97**
 trials 40–41
foot-and-mouth disease 102
forage mites 50
fungal cultures 59, 63, 111
fungal diseases 59, 82–89
fungi 14, 15, 88
furunculosis 69

genitalia, habronemiasis 54, 55
ghost figures 85, **87**
Giemsa stain 68, 83
glanders 91
glucocorticoids 15, 19, 23, 97
 Culicoides 46
 dependence 24
 immunosuppression 102
 insect allergy 96
 pruritus 21, 22, 40
 systemic 19, 37
 topical 19, 20, 37
 urticaria 43
 vasculitis 114
GMS 14
Gram stain 68

granulomas, eosinophilic 35, 92–93, **93**
grasses 40
gray horses 119, 122, **123**
Gridley stain 83
grooming tools 69
groundnut allergy 2, **8**

Habronema 1, **6**, 46, 99
 infection **92**, 116–117, **116**
  diagnosis 56
  face 54, **55**
  pastern 54, **55**
  ulcers **101**
 majus 54, 91
 muscae 54, 91
habronemiasis 1, 99
 crusts **9**
 cutaneous 54–57, 91–92
 eyes 54, **54**
 fly control 57
 genitalia 54, **55**
 healing stages **93**
 histopathology 56, **56**, 57
 lower legs 116–117
 prednisolone 92
 tissues 56, **56**
 treatment 56–57
 ulcers **9**, 10
 wound care 57
Haematobia irritans 47
Haematopota spp. 47
hair
 follicles 105, 107
 shaft morphology 13–14
Hematopinus asini 51
herpes 121–122
histamine reaction 15
Histoplasma 90
 capsulatum 85
histoplasmosis 85
history 1–3
hives 2, 6, 7, 21, 35, **36**, 42–43, **42**
horn flies 47
horse flies 47
humid climate 32, 46
humoral response 62
hydrocortisone 20, 37
hydroxyzine 15, 22, 38
hyperesthetic leukotrichia 121
hyperkeratosis 9, 11, **11**, 115
hyperpigmentation 3, 9–10, **11**, 110, 119
hypersalivation 101, **101**
hypersensitivity *see Culicoides* hypersensitivity
hypoallergenic shampoos 19
hypopigmentation 3, **11**, 119–123
hyposensitization, subcutaneous injection
  39–40, *40*

Mucorales 89
multidrug resistance 23
multisystemic eosinophilic epitheliotropic disease 74, **75**, **76**
mycetoma, eumycotic 88
Mycobacterium spp. 14
mycoses, deep 84–85
mycosis fungoides 63

Namibian horses, reticulated leukotrichia 121, **122**, **123**
necrotizing dermatitis 102
neem oil 37
nematodes 52–57, 91–92
neoplastic diseases 12, 93
neutrophils 63, 99
niacin 15
Nocardia spp. 14
nodular dermatitis 15, 82, **83**
nodular diseases 82–95, *83*
nodules 5, **6**, 14
    bacterial diseases 89–91
    differential diagnoses 12
    fungal diseases 82–89
    infectious causes 82–92
    parasitic diseases 91–92
    sterile inflammatory causes 92–93
non-follicular pustular diseases 59

oatmeal 20, 37, 42
occult sarcoids 76–77, **78**
Onchocerca 46, 52, **53**, 54
    cervicalis 52
    volvulus 3
onchocerciasis 3, 52–54, **53**
oomycetes 85
oomycotic infections 85–88
orthokeratosis 11
otitis 50
Otobius megnini 51
oxychlorine 21, 47, 62

Palomino horses 105
papillomavirus 75, 93
papules 4, **4**, 11, 60, **61**, 65
parasites 1, 21, 46–57, 59, 91–92
PAS 14
pastern 96
    dermatitis
        Chorioptes 112, **112**
        clinical approaches 110–118
        diagnostic work-up *111*
        differential diagnoses 111
        draft horses 110
        insects 112
        lymphedema 115–116, **116**
        predisposing factors 110, *111*
        shampoos 112
        skin biopsy 111

        skin scraping 111
        vasculitis **113**, **115**
    dermatophilosis 66, **66**
    Habronema infection 54, **55**
    Pythium lesions 85, **86**
Pasteurella spp. 90
patch test 16, **17**, **18**
Pediculoides ventricosus 50
pemphigus
    foliaceus 14, 59, 70–74, 79, 96,
           115–116, **115**
        alopecia 71, **71**
        azathioprine 73–74
        coronary band **72**
        cytology 72
        dexamethasone 72
        diagnosis 72
        draft horses 2
        histopathology 72, **73**
        pigmentation 119, **121**
        prednisolone 72, 73
        pustules 70–71, **70**
        skin biopsy 72
        treatment 72–74
        vaccination **71**, 72
    vulgaris 100–101
penicillin 2, 23
pentoxifylline 22–23, 42, 113, 114
permethrin 36, 47, 51, 112
phaeohyphomycosis **4**, 88–89, **89**
phosphatidylcholine 20
photosensitization **68**, 98, **98**, **99**, **100**, 113
physical examination 3
picaridin 36
pigeon breast 90
pigmentary changes, clinical approach 119–123
pigmentary incontinence 120
pigmentation 17, 119, **121**
    factors 119–120, *120*
plaques 5, **6**, 12
pollen 24, 38, 39, 113
    allergy 32, 33, 43
polymerase chain reaction (PCR) 68
post-inflammatory depigmentation **12**
potassium
    hydroxide 14
    iodide 85
poultry mites 50
pramoxine 20
prednisolone 22, 37, 54, 72, 73, 76,
    92, 93
pregnancy 62
pressure sores 103
primary lesions 3, 4–7
primary seborrhea 59
proactive therapy 20
probiotics 23, 37

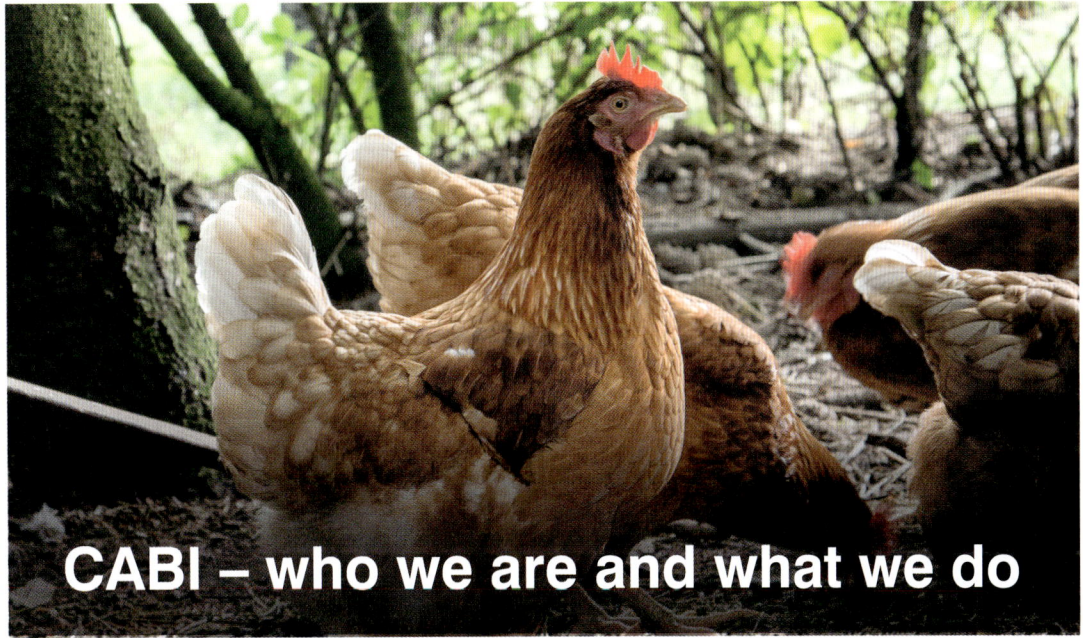

CABI – who we are and what we do

This book is published by **CABI**, an international not-for-profit organisation that improves people's lives worldwide by providing information and applying scientific expertise to solve problems in agriculture and the environment.

CABI is also a global publisher producing key scientific publications, including world renowned databases, as well as compendia, books, ebooks and full text electronic resources. We publish content in a wide range of subject areas including: agriculture and crop science / animal and veterinary sciences / ecology and conservation / environmental science / horticulture and plant sciences / human health, food science and nutrition / international development / leisure and tourism.

The profits from CABI's publishing activities enable us to work with farming communities around the world, supporting them as they battle with poor soil, invasive species and pests and diseases, to improve their livelihoods and help provide food for an ever growing population.

CABI is an international intergovernmental organisation, and we gratefully acknowledge the core financial support from our member countries (and lead agencies) including:

 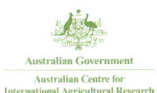 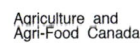 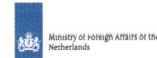 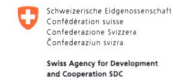

Discover more

To read more about CABI's work, please visit: **www.cabi.org**

Browse our books at: **www.cabi.org/bookshop**,
or explore our online products at: **www.cabi.org/publishing-products**

Interested in writing for CABI? Find our author guidelines here:
www.cabi.org/publishing-products/information-for-authors/